Life After Brain Injury

This is the first book of its kind to include the personal accounts of people who have survived injury to the brain, along with professional therapists' reports of their progress through rehabilitation. The paintings and stories of survivors combine with experts' discussions of the theory and practice of brain injury rehabilitation to illustrate the ups and downs that survivors encounter in their journeys from pre-injury status to insult and post-injury rehabilitation.

Wilson, Winegardner and Ashworth's focus on the survivors' perspective shows how rehabilitation is an interactive process between people with brain injury, health care staff and others, and gives the survivors the chance to tell their own stories of life before their injury, the nature of the insult, their early treatment and subsequent rehabilitation.

Presenting practical approaches to help survivors of brain injury achieve functionally relevant and meaningful goals, *Life After Brain Injury: Survivors' Stories* will help all those working in rehabilitation understand the principles involved in holistic brain injury rehabilitation and how these principles, combined with theory and models, translate into clinical practice.

This book will be of great interest to anyone who wishes to extend their knowledge of the latest theories and practices involved in making life more manageable for people who have suffered damage to the brain. *Life After Brain Injury: Survivors' Stories* will also be essential for clinical psychologists, neuropsychologists and anybody dealing with acquired brain injury whether they be a survivor of a brain injury themselves, a relative, a friend or a carer.

Barbara A. Wilson is a neuropsychologist and founder of the Oliver Zangwill Centre for Neuropsychological Rehabilitation in Ely, UK. She has worked in brain injury rehabilitation for over 35 years and has published 18 books, 270 journal articles and chapters and 8 neuro-psychological tests. Among her many awards she has an OBE and two lifetime achievement awards. She is the editor of the journal *Neuropsychological Rehabilitation* and has a rehabilitation centre in Ecuador named after her.

Jill Winegardner is a clinical neuropsychologist with 30 years' experience in brain injury assessment and rehabilitation. She has worked in a range of settings including acute inpatient, acute and post-acute rehabilitation, residential rehabilitation and outpatient care. She is currently lead clinical psychologist at the Oliver Zangwill Centre for Neuropsychological Rehabilitation. Her clinical and research interests include neuro-psychological assessment and rehabilitation, and programme design and evaluation.

Fiona Ashworth is a clinical psychologist with over ten years' experience working with people with acquired brain injury. Since completing her doctorate in clinical psychology at the University of Oxford, she has worked for five years at the Oliver Zangwill Centre for Neuropsychological Rehabilitation. She is currently a senior lecturer in Psychology at Anglia Ruskin University. Fiona also continues to work as a clinical psychologist at the Evelyn Community Head Injury Service, a project developed by the Oliver Zangwill Centre.

Life After Brain Injury

Survivors' Stories

Barbara A. Wilson, Jill Winegardner and Fiona Ashworth

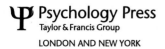

Psychology Press
Taylor & Francis Group
LONDON AND NEW YORK

First published 2014
by Psychology Press
27 Church Road, Hove, East Sussex BN3 2FA

Simultaneously published in the USA and Canada
by Psychology Press
711 Third Avenue, New York, NY 10017

*Psychology Press is an imprint of the Taylor & Francis Group,
an informa business*

British Library Cataloguing in Publication Data
A catalogue record for this book is available from the
British Library

Library of Congress Cataloging in Publication Data
Wilson, Barbara A., 1941–
Life after brain injury : survivors' stories / Barbara Wilson,
Jill Winegardner, Fiona Ashworth.
pages cm
1. Brain damage — Patients — Rehabilitation — Case
studies. 2. Brain damage — Patients — Rehabilitation —
Biography.   Head — Wounds and injuries — Therapists
and patient — Case studies. I. Winegardner, Jill,
1953– II. Ashworth, Fiona, 1977– III. Title.
RC387.5W547 2013
617.4 '81044 — dc23

                                        2013014397

ISBN: 978–1–84872–111–1 (hbk)
ISBN: 978–1–84872–112–8 (pbk)
ISBN: 978–0–203–37031–5 (ebk)

Typeset in Times New Roman
by RefineCatch Limited, Bungay, Suffolk

Printed and bound in the United States of America by Publishers Graphics,
LLC on sustainably sourced paper.

As I rise from the ashes of my broken former self,
I wonder where this torrid and unknown skyline is
    leading me?
Uncertainly, I spread my wings and start to rise up,
My wings start to gain momentum and I feel strong
    and free again!
In the distance I can see a small, white snowdrop.
Its simplicity and purity is beautiful and draws me
    to it,
Transmitting hope.

By Natalie Barden (Chapter 3)

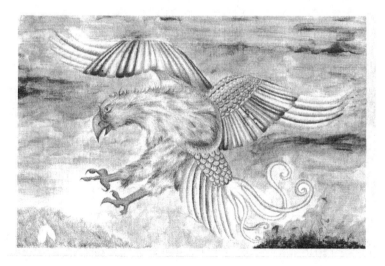

Natalie's Understanding Brain Injury project: The phoenix rising from the ashes.

Contents

Illustrations

Figures

Table

Foreword

Andrew Bateman

In a previous foreword to an earlier book by Barbara A. Wilson and colleagues, Keith Cicerone was quoted as saying, 'The goal of rehabilitation, to assist people to lead meaningful, fulfilling lives, is a tremendous undertaking, one that cannot be accomplished without a true collaborative effort.' The quotation seems even more appropriate for this book, which includes original accounts by survivors of head injury of their passage through trauma, rehabilitation and survival as well as descriptions and reports of the work completed by neuropsychologists and allied professionals on behalf of and in cooperation with those survivors. The book is both innovative and possibly unique in giving voice to the survivors themselves: the reader is thereby given a three-dimensional perspective, as it were, on rehabilitation after brain injury; the thoughts and feelings of clients are presented, as well as the objective reporting by therapists describing the same events and procedures.

The stories presented in this book encompass many restrictions to functioning: physical, emotional, social, cognitive and vocational aspects of life are included. Throughout a broad range of disabilities are some unifying themes of complexity, identity and relationships. The individuals go beyond *surviving* and are able to inform us about the potential to overcome the consequences of acquired brain injury, to live new if altered lives. We gain insights into the meaningfulness of the endeavour of providing rehabilitation by both clients and the professionals working with them.

A good clinical assessment should create a record of the experience of people who are seeking to overcome brain injury and makes for a good starting point. We certainly get this from the three authors whose expertise in brain injury rehabilitation is compellingly obvious from their professional assessments, observations, records and recommended treatments. Added to this, we have each survivor's detailed feedback and narrative, and in many cases the added reportage from their families. The in-depth patient reports here provide an indication of the landscape that needs to be covered when considering quality of life after brain injury. After ten years as manager at the Oliver Zangwill Centre (OZC), it gives me great pleasure to reflect on the chapters that are examples of the successes that have been achieved by our clients. Many of those treated at the OZC were treated free of charge under the National Health Service of the United Kingdom, and the state-of-the-art treatment thereby provided should be noted and applauded.

I remain filled with admiration for the clinicians who skilfully engage with these life stories to help people develop their goals and sense of agency. To write about your clinical work is a demanding task that requires effort over and above the routine day-to-day duties of assessing and providing therapy. Barbara, Fi and Jill have put many hours into this book to make it a reality. I am thankful for this because these are stories that need to be told. Most of all, I admire the determination and bravery of the individuals who have experienced the most isolating experience, described as a 'threat to self'. Their willingness to participate in sharing these stories is something for which I am extremely grateful.

Andrew Bateman, Clinical Manager, The Oliver Zangwill Centre for
Neuropsychological Rehabilitation
January 2013

Preface

It is possible that this book is unique in that it has been written by a very close team consisting not only of neuropsychologists from the same institution, but also their clients and patients. While it can be extremely difficult for survivors of brain injury to tell their stories as they may have to re-live traumatic events, those who have contributed so vitally to this book have captured the stress of their accident or illness, their journey through rehabilitation and their emergence from the dark times to lead meaningful lives. We cannot thank them enough for agreeing to join with us in this venture.

We expect readers of this book will consist in the main of professionals working in neuro-rehabilitation, other survivors of brain injury and their families, and purchasers of health care. However, we hope that the book will appeal to the general reader who may know very little about the effects of brain injury apart from headline news in the media, which is here today and gone tomorrow. We have included some technical detail and references that you might want to overlook if they are not relevant to your reading. By reading the book we anticipate readers will obtain the fullest picture of what it is like to sustain an insult to the brain and what can be done afterwards for survivors. It is our hope that the descriptions, analyses and explanations will clarify many issues involved in brain injury rehabilitation. Readers will learn that while we do not anticipate our clients recovering to their pre-injury state, we do plan for and expect them to lead a purposeful and reasonably fulfilling life.

We are aware that not everyone is able to achieve as successful an outcome as many of the people in our book have done. So many factors influence outcome: funding, timing, the right rehabilitation for the kind of injury experienced, external supports and more. If this is true for you, your family member or your client, we hope some of these stories will give you food for thought and new energy to seek the services the survivor deserves. At the same time we caution that the strategies and techniques described here should only be tried with the support of a trained rehabilitation professional.

Acknowledgements

We first wish to thank Rachel Winson for her extremely thoughtful and detailed editorial review. She not only used her excellent writing skills and publishing experience to offer insights that have greatly improved the original manuscript, she was also one of the OZC occupational therapists whose clinical skills contributed to good outcomes. We are very grateful to Mick Wilson for his practical support, brainstorming with us and help with proof reading. A special thanks is due to Wes Anderson for his support and patience and for walking Tonka while Fi worked on the book. Many thanks to Judy Butler for her editing assistance and bringing the fresh eyes of an outsider to her review. And a special thank you to Andrew Bateman, Clinical Manager of the OZC, for his time and dedication to the service.

We thank Catherine Tunnard for typing Claire's handwritten notes, Bonnie-Kate Dewar for her work with Claire, Patricia Montañes for putting us back in touch with Jose David, Jonathan Evans for his support with Mark and Jose David, Richard Greenwood for going above and beyond in supporting Mark, Huw Williams for assistance with Mark, Gerhard Florschutz for permission to write the stories of Tracey and Christine, and Angela Hinchcliffe for all her help with Tracey and Christine. Finally, a big thank you to all the non-OZC therapists and health professionals who also worked with these survivors.

We wish to acknowledge the tremendous contributions of the clinical team, past and present, from the Oliver Zangwill Centre, whose caring creativity and dedication to the practice of holistic neuropsychological rehabilitation have made possible these stories. Endless thanks to Anna Adlam, Judith Allanson, Andrew Bateman, Leah Bousie, Sue Brentnall, Rob Brindley, Stella Chan, Alexis Clarke, Joe Deakins, Rory Devine, Jane Emerton, Catherine Ford, Fergus Gracey, Louise Higgins, Jessica Ingham, Caroline Jennings, Clare Keohane, Lambchop the Therapy

Dog, Emma Louch, Donna Malley, Siobhan Palmer, Philippa Powell, Leyla Prince, Kate Psaila, Becky Rous, Maria Saez Martin, Carolyne Threadgold, Chantel Williams and Rachel Winson.

We thank our fabulous admin team for their hard work behind the scenes supporting clients with transport, accommodation and much more. Thanks to Liz Bush, Rachel Everett, Donna Johnson, Sharon McEwing, Amy Rideout and Michelle Young.

We are grateful to Taylor & Francis for permission to reproduce the model in Chapter 1 (Wilson, B. A. (2002). Towards a comprehensive model of cognitive rehabilitation. *Neuropsychological Rehabilitation*, *12*, 97–110).

And finally, we acknowledge the families of our survivors, whose lives were also indelibly altered by the events affecting their loved ones. Brain injury is indeed a family affair.

Chapter I

Introduction

Barbara A. Wilson

Unlike damage to a limb or indeed even another organ, damage to the brain can be debilitating to an extent that those injured remain dependent on others for the rest of their lives. Except in rare circumstances, a brain cannot be substituted by an artificial device or treated back to its original form or capacity, so brain injured people have to learn how to live their lives with handicaps that are not going to disappear over time.

In recent times workers in the field of neuro-rehabilitation have built up an extensive knowledge of the consequences of injury to the brain, they have developed sophisticated ways of analysing and diagnosing problems faced by brain injured people, and they have developed scientifically supported methods of treatment. The neuropsychologists who have contributed to this book have been able to draw upon an extensive literature of research and treatment as well as their own experiences in the field of brain injury rehabilitation. We stress again, however, that what makes this book unique is that the team of authors has been extended to include brain injured survivors themselves, thereby providing as full an account of brain injury and its consequences as possible. We are fairly confident that this book goes deeper and further than most if not all other books describing case studies dealing with the effects of brain injury, which rarely if ever include the story from the patient's point of view, and that barely touch upon the intricacies and efforts involved in brain injury rehabilitation.

There is much misunderstanding about the nature and consequences of brain injury and unfortunately this sometimes extends into the professional community and even exists among medical and political authorities who ought to know better! It is far too easy for some in authority, who do not wish to use some of the funds for which they are responsible, to accept that once a person can walk out of a hospital nothing else needs to be done. This is rarely the case for someone who has received an insult

to the brain. Holders of the country's purse strings can easily be seduced
by modern technology, preferring to spend money on machines that can
light up colours in the brain but cannot as yet indicate treatment for the
individuals whose brains light up! Meanwhile professionals working in
neuro-rehabilitation are starved of funding despite the fact that brain
injured people are convincingly helped to lead better daily lives after
receiving treatment at the hands of clinical and neuropsychologists,
occupational therapists and speech and language therapists. The irony is
that brain injured people who do not receive the sort of rehabilitation
described in this book can ultimately become a much larger financial
burden upon the state. Rehabilitation not only makes life better for brain
injured patients and their families, it also makes economic sense.

There is evidence to show that rehabilitation may be expensive in
the short term but it is cost effective in the long term (Prigatano &
Pliskin, 2002; Winegardner & Ashworth, 2012). There are several
studies suggesting that rehabilitation for survivors of brain injury
is economically effective. For example, Cope et al. (1991) surveyed
145 American patients and found that the estimated saving in care costs
following rehabilitation for a person with severe brain injury was over
£27,000 ($40,500) per year. The number of people requiring 24 hours
per day care dropped from 23% to 4% after rehabilitation. A Danish
study (Mehlbye & Larsen, 1994) reported that expenditure in health and
social care for patients attending a non-residential programme were
recouped in five years. The costs of not rehabilitating people with brain
injury are considerable given the fact that many are young with a
relatively normal life expectancy (Greenwood & McMillan, 1993). Cope
(1994) suggests that post-acute rehabilitation programmes can produce
sufficient savings to justify their support on a cost–benefit basis.

On a slightly different theme, a study by West et al. (1991) claimed
that people with traumatic brain injury (TBI) who had attended a
supported work programme earned more than the programme costs after
58 weeks of supported employment. Furthermore, after two and a half
years there was a net gain to the taxpayers who had ultimately funded the
service. This did not include the indirect costs such as savings from
family members who were able to return to work. Indirect costs have
also been reported by Teasdale et al. (2009), who found that the strain
on caregivers was reduced following use of a pager to remind patients
what to do. Wood et al. (1999) wanted to establish the clinical and
cost-effectiveness of a post-acute neurobehavioural community rehabilitation programme provided for 76 people surviving severe brain injury.
The majority had sustained their injuries more than two years prior to

admission and all had spent at least six months in rehabilitation. In terms of improved social outcomes and savings in care hours, it was found that the most cost-effective benefit was the provision of rehabilitation within two years of head injury; and it was still worthwhile, in terms of clinical and cost-effectiveness, to offer rehabilitation to those who were more than two years post-insult. Not only can rehabilitation save lives and improve quality of life for people with brain injury, it can also lead to major savings for government systems. It is estimated that people with moderate to severe brain injuries will have health and social care service costs of between £20,000 and £40,000 per year. A 25-year-old denied rehabilitation of the kind described in this book, and who lives to 75 years, may accrue costs of between £1,000,000 and £2,000,000. There is plenty of evidence to show that comprehensive neuropsychological rehabilitation is clinically effective. Cicerone and his colleagues, for example, in a meta-analysis, found that such programmes can improve community integration, functional independence and productivity, even for patients who are many years post injury (Cicerone et al., 2011). Van Heughten, Gregório and Wade (2012) looked at 95 randomised control trials carried out between 1980 and 2010 and concluded that there is a large body of evidence to support the efficacy of cognitive rehabilitation.

Rehabilitation for people with brain injury, conducted by qualified experts, is complex and demanding of expertise. It is not simply a tag on to medical treatment; neither is it in any way less complicated than analysing the results of MRI scans. We hope to show this in the following pages, and initially I would like to present a framework for rehabilitation that I developed a few years ago (Wilson, 2002) showing the areas that need to be considered and negotiated in order to provide effective treatment to brain injured individuals (see Figure 1.1). Obviously, not all areas will apply to each of the clients in this book. However, when contemplating each treatment described, the reader should be able to recognise particular pathways through the framework. At the end of this book we return to the framework to ask the reader whether we have kept to these pathways and been able to reach any kind of successful destinations as far as the clients are concerned.

The starting point for any rehabilitation programme is the patient or client and his or her family. In addition to background and ethnic and social issues, the nature, extent and severity of brain damage should be determined. Current problems, including cognitive, emotional, psychosocial and behavioural, need to be assessed. Models of language, reading, memory, executive functioning, attention and perception are available to

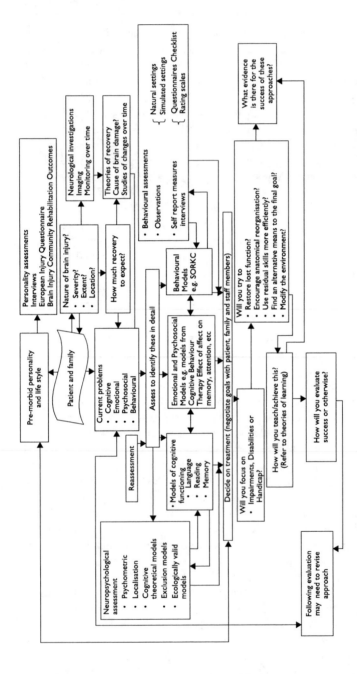

Figure 1.1 A model of Neuropsychological Rehabilitation (Wilson 2002, reproduced with permission of Taylor & Francis/Psychology Press).

provide detail about cognitive strengths and deficits. We can use assessment tools to determine emotional, behavioural, and social difficulties. Behavioural or functional assessments can be used to complement standardised assessment procedures. Having identified problems, the rehabilitation programme can be planned. Patients, families, and staff need to negotiate meaningful, functionally relevant, and attainable goals. Ways to achieve these goals need to be formulated (for example through compensatory techniques or through particular learning strategies). Whichever method is selected, theories of learning need to be consulted, understood and applied where necessary. In Baddeley's words, 'A theory of rehabilitation without a model of learning is a vehicle without an engine' (Baddeley, 1993, p. 235). It is now accepted that social, emotional, and cognitive functions are interlinked and difficult to separate (Wilson, Gracey, Evans & Bateman, 2009), so we should be aware of models of therapeutic change such as therapeutic working alliance, or the client's experience of being understood, which optimise learning and engagement in rehabilitation. Recent theories of identity (Gracey & Ownsworth, 2008), Compassion Focused Therapy (CFT; Ashworth, Gracey & Gilbert, 2011) and Narrative Therapy (White & Epston, 1990) are some of the latest additions to our treatment approaches.

As part of the complete process of rehabilitation, our treatments or interventions must be evaluated. Whyte (1997) pointed out that outcome should be congruent with the level of intervention. If intervening at the impairment (body structure and process) level then outcome measures should be measures of impairment and so forth. As most rehabilitation is concerned with the improvement of social participation, outcome measures should reflect changes in this domain: for example, how well does someone who forgets to take medication now remember to take medication? We are continuously improving our evaluation of neuropsychological programmes but it is not easy. As Hart, Fann and Novack (2008) remind us, because of the great heterogeneity of patients receiving such rehabilitation and because of the variety of aims and methods required to achieve ultimate goals, the measurement of treatment effectiveness and final outcomes resulting from rehabilitation are difficult to evaluate (Hart et al., 2008).

When considering the model, it is not difficult to recognise the labyrinth of theories to be negotiated in order to design treatment that is appropriate for each brain injured individual with his or her particular needs. The same is true when considering the circumstances and needs of that person's family and even in some cases the wider community. We have made considerable progress in recent times (Cicerone *et al.*, 2011) and are better at linking theory and practice (Wilson *et al.*, 2009) when designing practical solutions for the management of the brain injured person's daily life. These practical solutions are discussed in each chapter and supported by theoretical underpinning. Despite considerable success, rehabilitation has to proceed with very limited resources. In some of the chapters, the survivors themselves comment on or allude to problems with funding. It is worth repeating once more that although rehabilitation for survivors of brain injury may seem to be expensive in the short term, it is cost effective in the long term. Given that most people who have survived an acquired brain injury and are referred for neuropsychological rehabilitation are young and will, on the whole, live a normal life span, they deserve to be given every chance to live as fulfilling a life as possible.

A major feature of the rehabilitation offered by the Oliver Zangwill team is its concentration on holistic treatment. A holistic approach to brain injury rehabilitation, 'consists of well integrated interventions that exceed in scope, as well as in kind, those highly specific and circum-scribed interventions which are usually subsumed under the term "cognitive remediation"' (Ben-Yishay & Prigatano, 1990, p. 40). The holistic approach was pioneered by Diller (1976), Ben-Yishay (1978) and Prigatano (1986). Ben-Yishay and Prigatano (1990) provide a model of hierarchical stages in the holistic approach through which the patient must work in rehabilitation. These are, in order: *engagement, awareness, mastery, control, acceptance* and *identity*. The holistic approach argues that it is futile to separate the cognitive, social, emotional and functional aspects of brain injury. Given that how we feel emotionally affects how we think, remember, communicate and solve problems, and also influences how we behave, we need to acknowledge that these functions are inter-connected, often hard to separate and all need to be dealt with in rehabilitation. Holistic programmes offer both group and individual therapy to increase awareness, promote acceptance and understanding, provide cognitive remediation, develop compensatory skills and provide vocational counselling.

Holistic programmes, explicitly or implicitly, tend to work through hierarchical stages, as described by Ben-Yishay and Prigatano (1990), and are concerned with:

(i) increasing the individual's awareness of what has happened to him or to her;
(ii) increasing acceptance and understanding of what has happened;

(iii) the provision of strategies or techniques to reduce cognitive problems;
(iv) the development of compensatory skills;
(v) the provision of vocational counselling.

All holistic programmes include both group and individual therapy. It can be argued that the holistic approach is less of a model and more of a series of beliefs, or, as Prigatano (1999) puts it, a series of 'Principles'. Nevertheless, it makes clinical sense and despite its apparent expense, in the long term it is probably cost-effective (Cope *et al.*, 1991; Mehlbye & Larsen, 1994; Wilson & Evans, 2002). In fact, there is mounting evidence that rehabilitation reduces the effect of cognitive, psychosocial and emotional problems, leading to greater independence on the part of the patient, reduction in family stress and eventual employability for many brain injured people (Cicerone *et al.*, 2005, 2011).

The programme at the Oliver Zangwill Centre (OZC) is based on these principles of holistic rehabilitation. Several chapters will refer to our assessment process and rehabilitation programme. Clients undergo assessment for programme suitability by attending the OZC for sessions with all team members that involve clinical interview, neuropsychological testing, mood assessment, family interview, community outings, functional tasks, participation in OZC meetings and lunch with current clients. Results are formulated as a poster that depicts the multiple contributions of personal and historic information, current context and the consequences of the injury on mood, cognition, communication and function.

The programme itself has evolved over time but essentially always includes attendance for 18 to 24 weeks with an intensive period devoted to psycho-education focused on themes including understanding brain injury, attention and memory, executive functions, communication and mood. Clients also learn and practise strategies dovetailed to their particular difficulties and receive individual psychological therapy to support them through the rehabilitation process. They then progress to the integration phase in which personal goals are developed and practised back in the client's own community. At present, clients attend the intensive phase for four days per week and the integration phase for two days per week, with follow up goal setting and reviews at three, six and twelve months post-discharge.

In their latest meta-analysis of neuropsychological rehabilitation, Cicerone and his colleagues (2011), as mentioned above, conclude that comprehensive holistic neuropsychological rehabilitation leads to improvement. They go even further in their guidelines when they say, 'Comprehensive-holistic neuropsychologic rehabilitation is recommended to improve post acute participation and quality of life after moderate or severe TBI' (Cicerone *et al.*, 2011, p. 526).

While this book is influenced by theory, it is the narrative of the survivors themselves that provides confirmation of the value of rehabilitation. White and Epston (1990) believe that stories or narratives shape a person's identity. Some of our survivors address this theme. We hope that their stories will help those working in rehabilitation to understand the principles involved in holistic brain injury rehabilitation and appreciate how these principles, combined with theoretical input, translate into clinical practice. In each chapter functionally relevant and meaningful goals, set by the therapist, the survivor and his or her family, are targeted; appropriate practical steps are taken; and outcomes evaluated. Finally, in acknowledging that rehabilitation is an interactive process between people with brain injury, health care staff and others, we give the survivors a chance to tell their own stories about their journey.

Chapter 2

Tim's story

A seemingly mild injury just waiting to be understood

Jill Winegardner and Tim Lodge

After a seemingly mild brain injury, this 52-year-old engineer found himself unable to work, alienated from his family and desperately unhappy. His key to success was learning to be compassionate towards himself, which allowed him to then use his cognitive strategies successfully. Now, he's back at work and his children feel as though they have their dad back.

Introduction

My name is Tim. I am 52 years old and I live in Cambridgeshire, UK with my wife, two children and our dog.

As a child in Cambridge, Tim rose to the top of his class. He was a studious young man who earned 98% on his science exams. Nevertheless, he left school at age 15 to work as a sheet metal worker, where he performed extremely well at the job. At age 23, Tim decided to take a year-long Bible school course and subsequently worked in a Christian mission as a mechanic. He spent several years combining work as a car mechanic with missionary work in Europe, where he met his German wife, Babs. The couple returned to England, where Tim earned a BSc in Design Engineering. He got a job starting on the shop floor but rose through the ranks to the position of Lead Design Engineer at the time of his injury. His work has involved the creative application of engineering to non-weaponry, novel military situations, for example creating a CT scanner that can be quickly set up in the desert, and designing security shelters. Prior to his injury, Tim was healthy, hard-working and devoted to his family.

Background of injury

My accident occurred in 2009, when I was knocked down while riding my bicycle home from work. After losing consciousness for a short time I was admitted to Accident and Emergency at Addenbrooke's Hospital. I was discharged two hours later but I had to return due to headaches and Bell's palsy. I was seen by the East Anglian Neurosurgery and Head Injury Service in September 2009 where I was diagnosed with severe post-concussion syndrome.

A CT scan at that time was read as normal, though there was a small right parietal non-displaced fracture in the skull.

Since the accident I had only returned to work for half a day. My headaches and fatigue did not allow me to work for longer than those four hours, something that was very frustrating for me. I tried to busy myself at home by doing DIY [do it yourself] tasks but often these would end up with angry outbursts when I made silly mistakes. As a designer of military equipment and having always worked in engineering I had excelled in simple DIY jobs and I did not understand why I was not capable of doing the simplest of tasks now. I had also never been someone who lost my temper, yet now I would snap at the slightest provocation. It seemed as if my brain had seized up. I even had difficulties in stringing a sentence together or remembering to do simple things like eat. Depression set in and I gradually retreated into myself.

My family had seen a big difference in me. I had changed from the easy-going family man into a moody, quick-tempered recluse. It affected my 10-year-old daughter hardest. She is on the Autistic Spectrum and struggled to make sense of why her Daddy had changed. She asked my wife, 'When will I get my Daddy back?' My wife told me how she would be scared to come close to me in case I lost my temper.

When seen in the Neurosurgery and Head Injury Service after his accident, Tim complained of ongoing but improving headaches and additionally of lethargy, difficulty with concentration, memory problems, anxiety and a short temper after the injury. Tim was seen again two months later with complaints of headache (improved), tinnitus, poor short-term memory and depression. He underwent neuropsychological assessment with results indicating low mood and impaired performance on tests of memory and learning. He was diagnosed with severe post-concussion syndrome (Sterr, Herron, Hayward & Montaldi, 2006).

By early 2010, Tim's situation had deteriorated, and he was avoiding social contact, experiencing ongoing cognitive and physical problems and hopelessness, had no structure to his day and had expressed suicidal ideation. He reported serious depression and anxiety, with considerable self-criticism. Of particular concern was an incident in which he had taken the dog for a walk in dark alleys in hopes of being attacked. He was referred urgently to the Oliver Zangwill Centre (OZC) in the hope of preventing further decline.

When Tim first came to us, he and his wife reported that as his initial awareness of difficulties increased, so did his level of distress. He had shown symptoms of post-traumatic stress disorder including frequent nightmares, social discomfort and isolation, panic attacks, general anxiety, and depression with suicidal thinking at one point. Once the depression was identified, Tim was started on anti-depressants and began psychotherapy. As a result, his mood lifted so that he was no longer actively suicidal. Nevertheless, he remained highly anxious, avoidant of social situations and very self-critical. His wife described him as a perfectionist who was very hard on himself for even minor perceived flaws.

Prior to his injury, Tim was perceived as the calm one in the family, showing endless patience with his children and helping his wife cope with their younger daughter's behavioural problems. They shared care of the children and he went to work at 6 or 6.30 am in order to come home when the children returned from school. Since the injury, Tim had been emotionally exhausted by his daughter's difficulties and struggled daily with irritability and managing his anger with her.

Babs said that her husband's loving kindness with the family had disappeared. He no longer communicated his emotions in an empathic way. Instead, his attitude could appear cold and callous, and he showed his temper and raised his voice. Babs thought her husband had the intention to project the kindness he used to show but could no longer do so. She described their marriage as previously strong and harmonious, and she missed the level of caring and intimacy they used to share.

Assessment

My first visit to the Oliver Zangwill Centre (OZC) was for an initial assessment where I met the cohort that was being treated at that time. It was fairly obvious that they had traumatic brain injury (TBI) and this made me uncertain that I was suitable for the programme. My injury was not immediately obvious and I was still not convinced that my diagnosis was accurate. My reasoning was that my fatigue, speech problems and forgetfulness were surely just the result of the shock and exhaustion. MRI scans had not shown any grey areas on my brain, casting doubts as to whether a brain injury had taken place.

During his Admissions Assessment, Tim reported moderate fatigue, poor sleep, daily headaches, tinnitus, blurry vision, diminished sense of smell and taste, and food cravings resulting in overeating and weight gain. Although he had many symptoms typical of post-concussion syndrome, his admission to the programme was almost scuppered by an experienced neuropsychologist who worried his problems were all psychological and thought that if we focused on the brain injury we would make things worse. Although not true in Tim's case, many people with neurologically mild injuries and litigation in process are seen as exaggerating their problems, either consciously or unconsciously. Instead of receiving appropriate rehabilitation, they are treated with suspicion and advised against treatment so as not to reinforce the 'false' diagnosis. We thought he had the complexity of physical, cognitive, emotional and functional symptoms that warranted intensive intervention.

Rehabilitation

Tim was admitted to the full rehabilitation programme. It was clear that fatigue management needed to be a part of Tim's programme so that he could tolerate the mental effort and full days that were required. Right at the beginning, he completed a fatigue diary and then a formulation of his fatigue to identify fatigue vulnerability factors, activities that tend to bring on fatigue, his experience of fatigue and the helpful or unhelpful responses that he might use to manage his fatigue (see Figure 2.1). Tim was aware that he tried to push on and ignore his fatigue, but he found various strategies including Goal Management Framework (GMF) (Duncan, 1986; Robertson, 1996) and compassionate mind training that were helpful for him.

On the first day of the programme I was introduced to the other four members of my cohort. It was natural that I would compare myself to these people to try and find common ground. We all had problems caused by traffic accidents, except one who had suffered a tumour on the brain. I was surprised at some of our common symptoms. This helped me as I still doubted my diagnosis and was wondering what the financial repercussions would be if I was not diagnosed with a brain injury.

I had fun bonding with the other 'clients' and with the staff, feeling a sense of security in their presence. We knew that if we made mistakes they would be genuinely accepted and this helped us put our guard down. We were not allowed to call ourselves 'stupid' when we tried but failed.

The therapeutic milieu is a major component of a holistic brain injury rehabilitation programme (Ben-Yishay, 2000; Wilson *et al.*, 2009). A

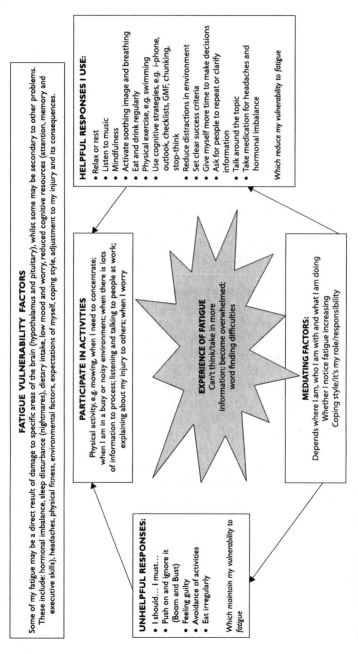

FATIGUE VULNERABILITY FACTORS

Some of my fatigue may be a direct result of damage to specific areas of the brain (hypothalamus and pituitary), whilst some may be secondary to other problems. These include: hormonal imbalance, sleep disturbance (nightmares), dietary intake, low mood and worry, reduced cognitive resources (attention, memory and executive skills), headaches, physical fitness, environmental factors, expectations of myself, coping style, adjustment to my injury and its consequences.

HELPFUL RESPONSES I USE:

- Relax or rest
- Listen to music
- Mindfulness
- Activate soothing image and breathing
- Eat and drink regularly
- Physical exercise, e.g. swimming
- Use cognitive strategies, e.g. i-phone, outlook, checklists, GMF, chunking, stop-think
- Reduce distractions in environment
- Set clear success criteria
- Give myself more time to make decisions
- Ask for people to repeat or clarify information
- Talk around the topic
- Take medication for headaches and hormonal imbalance

Which reduce my vulnerability to fatigue

PARTICIPATE IN ACTIVITIES

Physical activity, e.g. mowing, when I need to concentrate; when I am in a busy or noisy environment; when there is lots of information to process; listening and talking to people at work; explaining about my injury to others; when I worry

EXPERIENCE OF FATIGUE

Can't think/take in more information; become overwhelmed; word finding difficulties

MEDIATING FACTORS:

Depends where I am, who I am with and what I am doing
Whether I notice fatigue increasing
Coping style/it's my role/responsibility

UNHELPFUL RESPONSES:

- I should.... I must...
- Push on and ignore it (Boom and Bust)
- Feeling guilty
- Avoidance of activities
- Eat irregularly

Which maintain my vulnerability to fatigue

Figure 2.1 Tim's fatigue formulation.

therapeutic milieu is the creation of an alliance among staff and clients in a group setting in which the clients experience trust and safety through constructive feedback as they develop an understanding of the consequences of their injuries and try out new strategies to compensate for them. Benefits include discovering they are not alone with their difficulties and learning from each other.

The programme introduced us to our brains as various sectors and explained what these parts are responsible for. Although I had never really been interested in my own physiology, I could not help but be fascinated by the explanations of what the results are when different parts of our brain or their connections are damaged. Realising that damage to some brain tissue would result in a particular effect would help me to rationalise and accept my brain injury. Tests at the hospital verified that my pituitary gland or its connections were damaged. The OZC staff surmised that due to my head suddenly rotating, the connections to the pituitary gland had probably been put under stress. This would give a good explanation as to how a gland located in the lower central part of my brain had been affected in the accident.

The first goal in holistic rehabilitation is Understanding Brain Injury. Tim found his symptoms to be confusing, scary and puzzling so it helped him to learn exactly how the brain works and how his own brain functions, and to put his changes in this perspective. The tests also verified that he truly had a brain injury, and this was comforting in helping him understand and accept his symptoms.

As part of this work Tim had sessions looking at his own and others' brain scans and developing an awareness of post-concussion syndrome and the difficulties that can occur after mild/moderate brain injury. He also learned about pituitary function, which was found to be reduced in his own case. Tim developed a brain injury project that contained information for other survivors of similar types of injury. He is hoping this will offer them both support and inspiration and that sharing his own personal experience will be of mutual benefit.

Tim's goals on entering the programme included: fatigue reduction; improving his post-traumatic stress, depression and anxiety; returning to work at a safe pace with the support of his employer; coping more effectively with his children and managing his emotional reactions; learning strategies to compensate for his neuropsychological impairments; and learning more about his brain injury. He also hoped to feel more comfortable in social situations and regain confidence and feel comfortable driving.

We were taught how to focus our minds on the important issues and when we forgot things, to try and find strategies to assist us. We learned how to avoid areas where we are likely to struggle and if we could not, how to prepare ourselves beforehand. We were given physical tasks to complete like cooking a meal for the staff. We had to purchase the food beforehand in a supermarket. One of us would be shovelling food into the wrong trolley while someone else would be duplicating purchases that had already been put in the trolley. This was all part of finding out how and when to apply our new armoury of techniques, sorting out the ones we found effective and learning to choose when and where to use them.

Our model of rehabilitation focuses on learning what the problems are, trying out various strategies to see what works, and then putting them into practice (Kolb, Boyatzis & Mainemelis, 2001). Tim is describing the use of behavioural experiments in which the clients take on practical tasks, predict how well they will do, receive encouragement to use the strategies they are learning, carry out the tasks and then reflect on how it went. This gives them an opportunity to pause and reflect (Stop–Think) and to process their experiences in a thoughtful and reflective way. This process of testing out ideas and reflecting on the experience helps build confidence and cement strategy use.

It was surprising to learn how the brain works. We found out that given enough concentration we could cut out even the obvious to allow our damaged brains to focus on the meaningful rather than the distractions that we all experience. This is now a daily part of my life and allows me to complete tasks that I struggled to complete before coming to the OZC. As a designer, I was used to having to manage myself so I could make creative decisions. Since the accident I had real difficulties in planning, preferring to look at the goal and somehow stumbling towards it as fast as I could. Sometimes this worked but at other times it would have disastrous consequences, often ending up in an uncompleted job and a major onset of depression.

Neuropsychological testing revealed that although Tim was a very bright man, he had mild impairment of attention, verbal learning and memory, and complex planning. His cognitive formulation can be found in Figure 2.2.

It seemed surprising to Tim how even apparently mild cognitive difficulties can result in constant and serious real-life problems.

Even in usual daily things like driving the car I would have difficulties. I smashed two tail-lights on the car on two different occasions on the same bush. I was trying to reverse into our driveway but because I did not focus on the problems that lay

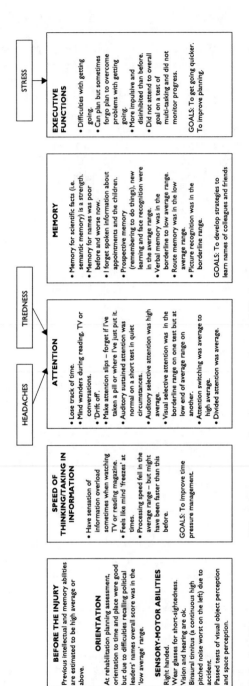

Figure 2.2 The consequences of Tim's brain injury: Cognitive strengths and difficulties.

in the way, I ended up with an expensive repair bill. Can you imagine what an idiot I felt like? I have driven buses up the small streets of London and now I cannot even park a car!

Tim found himself being highly self-critical and then losing self-confidence. His reaction to the cognitive difficulties he was experiencing highlights the fact that cognitive problems and emotional reactions are highly intertwined. Tim's comments are a good illustration of the way in which self-critical people are extremely sensitive to even small errors and then beat themselves up. When the cognitive problems are misunderstood or trivialised by oneself or others, serious self-doubt and subsequent self-criticism are even more likely.

Once I had been taught Goal Management Framework (GMF), I started to apply it even to small tasks such as parking. It went a little like this:
What do I want to do? Park the car in drive.
Clarify. I want to reverse the car into the driveway without driving over the neighbour's cat, hitting other cars, the garage door or the bush and at a safe pace. I then want to secure it and leave it suitably positioned so the next user will not have any difficulties getting in the car or manoeuvring it out of the parking space.
Is there only one solution? No. I could (a) spend more time on manoeuvring the car into the space, perhaps with help from someone else or (b) I could chop down the bush, widen the driveway and cone off the road by my parking space.
Evaluate solutions. Well it is obvious is it not?
Carry out plan.
Overall evaluation: Well since the bush is not there anymore it is soooo much easier to park.

The GMF is described in Figure 2.3 entitled 'My Cognitive Strategies', along with other strategies that Tim learned during the intensive phase of the programme.

During the first six weeks of the course, we had a week on communication. This was a strong point of mine before the accident; after all, I had to communicate the information of my design in a number of different ways so that my customers, peers and production workers could understand clearly what I was proposing as a design. After the accident I found it hard to communicate due to word-finding problems and a deficiency to focus my attention for longer periods. My self-confidence fell and my depression was exacerbated as I was aware of the difficulties I was having speaking to others. People I knew would be more understanding (although they would often start replying while I was still mid-sentence). Talking with strangers was avoided at all costs.

My Cognitive Strategies

SPEED OF THINKING/TAKING IN INFORMATION	ATTENTION	MEMORY	EXECUTIVE FUNCTIONS
TIME PRESSURE experienced when: - finishing a design - at design review meetings - given unexpected tasks - giving presentations - completing a 'to do' list of tasks at home	**STRATEGIES:** **USE MY ATTEN-TION BEAM** by being aware and in control of what I'm focusing on **TAKE BREAKS** **MANAGE DISTRACTIONS** both internal and external	**STRATEGIES:** **CREATE REFERENCE SHEETS OF KEY INFO** To verify memories when it's important to be accurate. - Only include key information. - Chunk information. - Link together key information (e.g. name, face, role). - Verify the information with someone else if possible. CHECK INFO ON STAND	**STRATEGIES:** **GMF for planning and problem solving** Use for all work tasks 1) Define goal. 2) Generate options. 3) Evaluate options. 4) Choose best option. 5) Plan steps to follow. 6) Monitor plan. **PRIORITISING BY URGENCY X IMPORTANCE** **'GETTING GOING' AT HOME** 1) Identify clear time for tasks. 2) Send myself texts/alerts to remind myself to start the task.
STRATEGY: TIME PRESSURE MANAGEMENT 1) Analyse task for time pressure (write out each step and tick those when I predict I'll feel under time pressure). 2) Prevent time pressure by doing steps/tasks beforehand where possible. 3) Plan how to handle unavoidable time pressure. 4) Monitor how my plan goes.			

Figure 2.3 Tim's cognitive strategies table.

Tim illustrates very well how cognitive problems, even milder ones, can impact on social participation. We saw his difficulties with word-finding as linked to areas such as reduced speed of processing and mood rather than the result of specific language impairment. This hypothesis gained support as the programme progressed, as Tim noted that communication was affected when he felt anxious or emotional. He became aware of the need to employ mood management strategies to aid his communication at these times.

During the communication week we were taught how to recall words or exchange words we were having difficulties with. We were taught how to be assertive and how to restrain ourselves rather than blurt out what was on our minds at inopportune moments. This instruction, together with the Mood Week, helped me rebuild my confidence in my ability to communicate.

The aims of the group were to identify and understand the skills involved in communication, to increase awareness of personal communication strengths and weaknesses and to have the opportunity to find out about different strategies and try these out in planned activities. In addition to this work, Tim continued communication work by exploring assertiveness and reframing communication accordingly. He was able to give work examples where he had utilised these skills and felt more confident as a result.

The Mood Week intrigued me, although at the start I was sceptical of how effective it would be. I could not understand how a psychological answer could apply to a physical problem. Indeed, when the psychologist started to talk about 'tricky' brains and how our tricky brains were not our fault I started to go on the offensive. She (the psychologist) talked about how our fight-or-flight mechanism in our brains is influenced by our 'old' and 'new' brains; our new brains governing the instinctive reaction (fight or flight) of our old brain. When asked for examples, I cited a case where in a moment of road rage I had lost my temper with another motorist. I asked if (had I hit the other motorist) when it came to court I could plead it was not my fault because my psychologist said I had a tricky brain! I do not think I was an easy client. I should mention that we were then taught how to take responsibility for any problems we may have inherited from our injuries. Those injuries may affect the breakdown in the function of the new brain controlling the old brain.

In Mood Week (based on a compassionate mind approach; see Gilbert, 2005, 2010a, 2010b) Tim learned that his emotional responses were partly due to the real losses and stresses going on but also to changes in the brain that govern our ability to monitor and regulate our emotions.

In fact I was greatly helped by the psychological side of the programme. Before I attended the centre, I had beaten myself up over every silly mistake I made (refer back to car parking problems for an example). I had always been very self-critical but the raft of really stupid mistakes that had occurred since the accident had left me with severe depression and doubting my self-worth. Being able to attribute these mistakes to the injury and learning how to implement techniques to stop them from happening again (or not as frequently) lifted a great load off my shoulders.

In Tim's rehabilitation, he learned both cognitive strategies to help him focus and plan better and emotional strategies that helped him calm and centre himself to be able to then use the cognitive strategies effectively.

In order to tackle self-criticism, anxiety, low mood and anger Tim was introduced to Compassion Focused Therapy (CFT) (Gilbert, 2005, 2010a, 2010b). He was encouraged to do some self-guided reading on CFT and to practise strategies of soothing rhythm breathing, safe place imagery and compassionate ideal imagery (e.g. imagery of an embodiment of compassion). Challenges to adopting a compassionate approach towards himself arose and were problem-solved in sessions. These led to the use of a photographic cue to aid compassionate ideal imagery in stressful situations and encouragement to be compassionate towards himself and others by not rushing to problem solve when feeling overwhelmed by other people's difficulties. Tim made strong gains early in therapy, for example, working out how to use his CFT techniques to take on cognitively and emotionally challenging tasks such as mending his car and driving for a longer journey than before. After building a strong base of CFT strategies, Tim was introduced to the technique of reviewing and updating traumatic memories from trauma-focused Cognitive Behavioural Therapy (Ehlers & Clark, 2000). With his therapist, Tim reviewed the thoughts and feelings associated with key traumatic memories and nightmares and updated these with new information (e.g. that he had not lost his job or home, that he retained the respect of others). At the end of the programme, Tim reported that the frequency of his nightmares had dropped from nightly to approximately three a week.

Over the next 12 weeks at the centre I would practise the techniques I had learned in the intensive phase. The protective environment and assistance that the staff gave me was a welcome break from going it alone. I learned to have compassion with myself when I lost my temper and when things got on top of me. It was a bit like walking a tightrope to start off with including lots of falls and much concentration. The team were always there to remind me of lessons learned and of past victories as well as helping me through some of the problems that were not covered in the main course. I was suffering from post-traumatic stress disorder (PTSD) which led to constant nightmares and panic attacks. This in turn would leave me exhausted with little energy to move on.

Many of these attacks centred on the fear of not being able to provide for my family and losing my successful career. With the help of the OZ team and a very supportive employer I started doing two days a week on reduced duties at work. One of the occupational therapists from OZ would meet regularly with my employer to ensure that I was properly catered for. They would address any problems and ensure that the rate of return and the workload was appropriate to my recovery.

For many people with brain injury, vocational rehabilitation is essential to allow a smooth and gradual return to work. As practice for presentations at work, Tim presented a critique of the Oliver Zangwill Centre at our daily community meeting. Working together with the therapist and the employer is optimal to ensure successful return to work. Tim and his therapist developed a summary and action plan.

VOCATIONAL SUMMARY AND ACTION PLAN

Summary of strengths:

- 100% attendance record while at OZC, including work trial days
- confident in ability to learn new tasks
- able to produce quality, accurate work
- willing to take on increased responsibility
- good use of initiative
- able to get along well with others
- responsive to feedback about performance
- understanding of the effects of my brain injury on my work performance

Summary of needs/strategies:

- Fatigue – I can manage this by using the GMF, taking breaks and eating/drinking regularly, listening to music, using my iPhone to organise my time efficiently.
- Brain freeze – I can manage this by talking around the subject, using repetition, taking a break.
- Memory – for semantic memory needs I can use my iPhone, white board, work computer.

- For working memory needs I can do checks, use the document stand next to my work computer.
- Speed of thinking – I can support this by using SQ3R (survey, question, read, recite, and review), taking breaks.
- Attention – I can support this by using the lighthouse technique (for directing one's attention), SQ3R, taking breaks, getting rid of distractions, using my mental blackboard.
- Planning – I can support this by using my whiteboard, iPhone (with home and work link), work computer.

To date I am doing 27 hours a week and I am performing above and beyond my own and my employer's expectations. I have confidence that I now have the clarity of mind to produce innovative ideas as I did before. Thanks to the help from OZC I am closer to the goals that I have to get back to work full-time and be a loving father/husband. I am aware that I will always have to live with the effects of a brain injury, but my youngest daughter no longer misses her old Dad and proves it by the hugs, wrestling matches and leap-frog competitions we have most evenings. I can help my eldest with her homework and I can support my wife rather than hide from the problems of family life.

Chapter 3

Natalie's story

The phoenix rising from the ashes

Fiona Ashworth and Natalie Barden

Natalie was a young woman with her whole life ahead of her. She was a 'free spirit', enjoying life with friends and family and seeing where life would take her. She was in love and looking forward to her future, until one fateful day at a music festival when a bleed on her brain changed her future forever.

Introduction

Thirty-four-year-old Natalie grew up in Cambridge with her family. She was a happy-go-lucky girl. When she finished school she went on to sixth form college and studied art history, art and English. After this she did an art foundation course and then she decided to train as a special effects make-up artist and work with foam latex and do model making. She soon realised how competitive this industry was and started working at a make-up counter in a large department store while she decided what to do next. While she enjoyed this, it was clear that Natalie was keen to challenge and stretch herself. She enjoyed socialising with her friends and had a keen interest in music and dancing. One night, Natalie was introduced to Ainsley by her brother. Although they had met before, there was a special spark they both felt that evening and this grew to a strong bond and friendship as they got to know each other. A year and a half later they became engaged when Natalie was in her early twenties.

Background of injury

Life was ticking along quite nicely; I just fancied doing something a bit different, having something to look forward to, maybe going away to do something a bit exciting. So, I suggested to my close friend, Beth, and my fiancé at the time, Ains, if they would like to go to Creamfields festival up in Liverpool to see Massive Attack, a band we all liked and wanted to see live.

I was 24 years old on August 24 2003, a date I will always remember, but when I woke up on that sunny morning with a dull ache in my right temple I had no idea the extent of things to come!

We had made our way down to the centre of Liverpool and had gone to a pub for lunch and a couple of drinks before heading to the Creamfields site, which was situated a bit out of town. I had taken some painkillers to try to get rid of the headache. We got there, and we were dancing, and I think I started to overheat and dehydrate. To make matters worse we spotted a stall selling herbal highs and decided to take a few of those, along with the vodka jellies and alcopops we were consuming, all in the name of a good time. Meanwhile my headache was still persisting and, if anything, getting more intense, and then it really started to pound, like a sickening thudding all over my head. As it was getting dark the pain began to get so intense it was turning my stomach and I felt incredibly sick, until in the end I was on my knees on the ground clutching my head in agony and throwing up because the pain was unbearable. I remember the dismay I felt as I heard the distinctive bass of Massive Attack's set beginning as I lay there on the grass unable to move, in agony, and I just thought, 'Oh bloody hell, I'm just ruining everyone's night!'

Things started to get hazy when I remember a little first aid truck with the profile of two people against a glowing, blinding white light as it made its way towards me. The next thing I remember is lying on my back on the floor of the first aid tent with a slightly cross woman with a clip board asking me questions in an offhand way. I really needed the toilet and so I asked her where the nearest one was. She pointed me in the right direction, I got up, and that was when I had the first seizure of my life. From this point on I have very little memory of what happened next except for surreal dream-like sequences that I would never know if they were part of my reality.

Natalie had suffered a stroke at age 24. She was admitted to hospital in Liverpool, where at the time her Glasgow Coma Scale (GCS) was 13/15, but this deteriorated to 9/15. She had a brain scan approximately 16 hours after the event. Hospital notes revealed that Natalie had suffered a spontaneous subarachnoid brain haemorrhage in the right fronto-parietal region. As a result of this, she underwent neurosurgery to evacuate an intracerebral haematoma, which almost killed her. Natalie had problems with life-threateningly high intracranial pressure and had a burr inserted. After she was stabilised she received neurorehabilitation as an inpatient at the Liverpool Hospital, which included physiotherapy and speech and language therapy. She was then sent home five weeks later.

Once I got home, that was when things became harder in lots of ways. Initially I was so glad to be back in our familiar environment, and to be with my fiancé in our flat, and to be able to see friends and family. The trouble was no one prepares you for how difficult it is going to be and how much your life changes. There was no real support available and we really found it hard to deal with everyday life. Ains had to give up work and of course I could not work because my left side and face was still paralysed and at this point it was still difficult for me to walk from one end of the room to the other as I was still getting my motor skills, and strength was returning slowly. Whilst I was in hospital I could hardly see, and the Optometrist there could not tell me if my sight would return or not. Luckily for me it improved slowly as time went on. I could now feed myself, mostly, and I had started to speak again, although it was very broken and like I was whispering! Money was tight but we had a lot of lovely visitors and I stared at a LOT of daytime TV!

Ains had applied for a flat with a housing society, which we got news about fairly quickly, and we were able to move in that February. By this time my motor skills had returned, and, although I was still suffering from fatigue very badly, things were ok, so I decided to try to go back to work part-time, this time based at Boots [pharmacy]. Looking back on this now, I did this too early as I couldn't cope, especially with all the standing, and we really struggled to manage with my now part-time wage. We did however get some gorgeous little kittens from Wood Green Animal Shelter, which made coming home from work a complete joy!

I tried the job for a good few months but it didn't work out, and I had to leave, which made me feel very depressed and worthless, but there was a slight sense of relief as it was very stressful. I took a bit of a break and then I had a go at a web design course but that was very complicated and too advanced for me, especially after a brain haemorrhage when memory and attention were an issue! Perhaps a touch unrealistic, I'm thinking now! I started volunteering at Headway (a charity for people with acquired brain injuries) around this time, which I really enjoyed. It was great working with service users who had a similar history to me, and knowing that I was helping in a small way was a wonderful feeling for me so I got a lot out of it.

After this I had a couple of part-time administrative jobs, although I didn't really enjoy them, but I thought it would be a 'suitable' idea as there was lots of that work around and I could sit down. But I found I was often battling against the side effects of my anti-convulsant medication to keep alert and to try not to feel so sleepy; either that or the awful headaches! The tablets, although I felt tired all of the time, would stop me from falling asleep so I would be exhausted, so there was rarely a happy medium with them! Meanwhile Ains and I were splitting up, which was awful and incredibly sad, but he wasn't coping with the way the haemorrhage had changed our lives, and me, and as much as I would have liked to have never had it happen I had to accept the person that I had become.

Then one day I saw an advert for a reception and photographic position with the university, which I got very excited about! I was delighted when I got a call to invite me in for an interview. It went well and I got the job and I was there for six years, until last year, but I was having some real problems again, partly to do with medication changes, and people being unwilling to make allowances for this. I started to have more seizures back in 2009 so my neurologist tried me on different anti-convulsants, but there is always an adjustment period with each medication and I've always found them to be very strong mind- and mood-altering drugs, which can affect your memory, energy levels and how or if you can sleep.

For those six years, Natalie grappled with trying to get her life back on track. As a result of her difficulties at work, in consequence of the stroke, Natalie was referred by her occupational health department to the Oliver Zangwill Centre (OZC). Aged 32, Natalie came for assessment in 2009 and we thought that she would benefit greatly from rehabilitation. However, due to funding issues she was unable to start rehabilitation, and it was estimated that she might need to wait another year before she could start the programme.

I started making mistakes at work, which my colleagues reported, and I was then called to the Assistant Staff Head of Department's office, and put onto a disciplinary, which made me feel even more stressed and terrible about myself! They eventually met with my union rep and arranged for me to be seconded to another department whilst I waited to hear about when I could start at the Oliver Zangwill Centre. The secondment arrangements were all done without consulting me, which, whilst I believe the intention was good, made me feel powerless and like I had no other choice. So, I started working two mornings a week in the other department with some really lovely people but doing soul-destroying work!

Unfortunately, the work situation worsened for Natalie and she became extremely depressed. She received funding to see a clinical psychologist at the OZC for psychotherapy at this time but she would still have to wait for the holistic rehabilitation programme.

I became really ill at this stage and extremely depressed. The anti-convulsant I was taking had been increased after I had a seizure on Boxing Day, then I'd had another one three weeks later so I was now taking 1200mg a day. I later found out a major side-effect of this drug was depression when the drug was taken in higher doses. I just felt like my existence was sucked into a black hole, I felt isolated, lonely, and that there just wasn't any point. It seemed to be raining all the time, and it was cold and grey, and a huge part of me just gave up and I lost my hope.

After this I went to live with Mum and Dad, and this was an incredibly difficult time for all of us as I was put on an anti-depressant medication, which made me obsessed with the idea of suicide, and I just felt stressed all of the time! Instead of making me feel happier and better, all I could look to was ending life and the relief of never having to worry about another tomorrow or that I would have to do or make plans. My hair was breaking off, I lost interest in food, I only ate when people reminded me and I could never finish what was on my plate as I never really wanted it, and my periods stopped. I became very thin and was totally convinced that the world would be a better place without me, and I desperately wanted to be gone and free so that I wouldn't be worrying anyone anymore! Just getting out of bed was a huge ordeal, or trying to go down the shop was extremely stressful and I'd actually get really scared and have to go with someone else so that they could protect me. I needed to have people around me as much as possible to distract me from the horrible thoughts going on in my head so I would arrange to meet up with friends for coffee, or they would come round as much as possible, or I would go out for walks with Mum. Rod, my Mum and Dad's friend, used to do yoga with me, which was great for trying to get strength back into my weakened body, and I used to talk to his wife Chris a lot and another lady called Sue who is a family friend. We would try to make sense of the hopelessness that was churning around in my head and in my heavy heart.

Natalie's mental health sadly deteriorated to the point that she felt she had no other option and she attempted suicide. She was hospitalised and then received input from the local community mental health team as well as from a private complementary medicine clinic. However, she still continued to struggle with the consequences of her stroke. She also continued to see our psychologist for psychotherapy for eight months prior to starting the rehabilitation programme.

I never thought I would be capable of doing the Oliver Zangwill Centre programme! I just thought I would be too tired all the time and too ill, my immune system was incredibly weak but it was a lot to do with my lack of self-confidence and self-belief as well. I thought I was totally worthless and incapable of anything! My programme was put back but I continued to have one-to-one sessions with my psychologist, which were very helpful, and then I began the programme in June.

Assessment

As is usual at the centre, Natalie saw all members of the holistic inter-disciplinary team to assess her rehabilitation needs. She met weekly with an occupational therapist (OT), psychologist, speech and language therapist (SALT) and an assistant psychologist.

Cognitive assessment

Neuropsychological assessment revealed difficulties with speed of processing, attention (including switching, dividing and sustained), prospective memory and executive functioning (making decisions and rigidity). Natalie herself reported slowed thinking, difficulties multi-tasking and particularly difficulties with sustaining and switching her attention between different things. She also noted forgetfulness and found it difficult to plan her time effectively to ensure she got things done on time.

Mood assessment

Natalie continued to work with the psychologist she had begun seeing for depression prior to starting the programme. The psychologist had worked with Natalie to improve mood, reduce suicidality and support Natalie so that she would be able to participate in the rehabilitation programme. Assessment at the start of the programme indicated that Natalie had low self-esteem, significant levels of anxiety, borderline symptoms of depression and high self-criticism, particularly expressed in a sense of inadequacy. Natalie also reported that since the brain injury she was lower in energy, lacking in contentment in herself and feeling lonely.

Speech and language assessment including social communication

Natalie's only difficulties in these areas were with flexible thinking and with describing her feelings as measured on the Toronto Alexithymia Scale (TAS) (Bagby, Parker & Taylor, 1994).

Functional assessment

Observation and assessment highlighted difficulties in day-to-day tasks consistent with findings from neuropsychological testing, including attentional and executive functioning difficulties, as well as slowed speed of processing. Fatigue monitoring also highlighted how Natalie's fatigue could impact on some activities. Vocational assessment using the Model of Human Occupation (Kielhofner, Braveman, Baron, Fisher, Hammel & Littleton, 1999) indicated that Natalie valued creativity and was keen to fulfil roles, including those of worker, home maintainer, friend and family member. Natalie described how she was struggling in her current job and not enjoying being there.

In summary, Natalie had multiple interacting cognitive and emotional difficulties, which were impacting on her ability to fully participate in her life.

Rehabilitation

Natalie attended a holistic neuropsychological rehabilitation programme. During the first six-week intensive phase, Natalie's rehabilitation needs and goals were assessed and she attended groups four days a week to increase her understanding of the consequences of her brain injury. During the second 12-week integration phase, Natalie focused on her personal goals, especially her wish to attain a greater understanding of the consequences of her brain injury so that she could develop strategies to overcome the impact of her difficulties on her everyday life.

Goal 1: Natalie will gain a clearer understanding of the cognitive, communication, mood and functional consequences of the stroke

Natalie achieved this goal through exploring her experiences in both group and individual sessions. She engaged well in the groups, and was observed to be a keen learner. It was clear that she was motivated, as she would often bring topics from the wider group relevant to herself to her individual sessions to clarify or learn more. As she gained a greater understanding of her key strengths and difficulties, Natalie was then able to begin exploring potential strategies to overcome difficulties.

Whilst I found it tiring being on the programme, it was wonderful, and I learnt so much about brain injury and myself and how hard I had been on myself as we learnt to exercise our compassionate selves again! Christine, the other lovely lady on the programme with me, and I developed a very close relationship. It is so helpful to meet other people who have experienced acquired brain injury, as it can feel so isolating. I also got a lot out of the group therapy sessions (Support Group) with the group who had come after us, and we worked through some really important issues together which were incredibly invaluable!

During the integration phase, Natalie focused on her personal goals in more depth, developing strategies for her needs. Her team had regular goal planning meetings to assure a shared understanding and coherent goal focus. Outlined below are the key goals pursued and the progress that Natalie made in each of these areas during the rehabilitation programme.

Goal 2: Natalie will practise Attention Training Techniques (ATT) to manage her attention

Natalie's top goal for cognitive work was to feel more in control of her attention. A shared understanding was developed of the broader cognitive difficulties, followed by a focus on the attentional component. Natalie described multiple everyday situations that were disrupted by her difficulties with attention, including doing tasks at work and remembering the content of conversations. Her attention difficulties had a clear emotional component, whereby rumination contributed to her anxiety and led to increased difficulties with attention. A perceived lack of control over attention reinforced these difficulties.

It was also evident that Natalie's difficulties with her attention were related to higher-level executive functions, which made it hard for her to encode information into memory. Natalie wanted a greater sense of control over her attention in everyday life, both with cognitive and emotional distracters. She was introduced to Attention Training Techniques (ATT) (Wells, 2008), which aim to improve flexible control over attention, particularly in relation to anxiety and depression but also in terms of focusing attention more generally. The training is aimed at working at a metacognitive level (Wells & Matthews, 1994), so we thought it would help Natalie not just with managing her attention in relation to emotional distracters but also with focusing her attention in non-emotive situations. She practised in cognitive sessions followed by reflection as well as daily practice outside of sessions. Gradually, Natalie started to generalise the ATT to everyday situations where she anticipated difficulties with her attention. We measured her success with ATT by using Wells' (2008) self-attention test as well as visual analogue scales (VAS) related to everyday life situations. Both measures showed positive changes in managing her attention.

Goal 3: Natalie will develop tools to aid memory, planning and time management

Natalie also developed compensatory strategies to aid memory and planning. As she was already successfully using a diary on entering the programme, we used this as the foundation upon which to build further strategies. Natalie learned the Goal Management Framework (GMF), a centre specific adaptation of Goal Management Training (GMT; Robertson, 1996), to facilitate everyday planning. Natalie found it difficult to plan under pressure, probably linked to her slowed speed of processing and attentional difficulties. Therefore, a behavioural experiment approach (Bennett-Levy, Westbrook, Fennell, Cooper, Rouf & Hackmann, 2004) was taken to test out various forms of the GMF and other compensatory approaches to planning, including Time Pressure Management (Winkens, Van Heugten, Wade, Habets & Fasotti, 2009).

This process was evaluated by asking Natalie to re-rate her confidence in completing tasks (with less sense of pressure) with and without planning strategies. By the end of the programme, Natalie had her own adapted tool for planning and time pressure management. She reported positive gains in effectiveness of the ATT and the planning tool. Overall, compared to the start of the programme, self-report measures of cognitive difficulties indicated a reduction in symptoms on both the European Brain Injury Questionnaire (EBIQ) (Sopena, Dewar, Nannery, Teasdale & Wilson, 2007) and the Dysexecutive Questionnaire (DEX) (Burgess, Alderman, Emslie, Evans & Wilson, 1996).

Goal 4: Natalie will learn to describe her emotions more effectively

Natalie's initial assessment indicated problems with alexithymia, which is difficulty recognising one's own emotions. Therefore, she wanted to develop her ability to describe how she was feeling. She worked with both her speech and language therapist and her psychologist to learn about and describe each of the six basic emotions through looking at photographs of her own face expressing emotions, giving examples of when she would express that particular emotion, noticing the physical response she experienced in relation to each of the emotions, and also looking at what external signs others might see on her face in order to understand how she was feeling. Natalie also monitored situations in which she experienced particular emotions over a number of weeks. She used Actiheart to monitor her heart rate responses to anger and anxiety and she kept a diary of situations in which she experienced the emotions. Alongside this work, psychotherapy sessions were also monitored by Natalie's psychologist to determine if her description of her emotions had changed.

Pre- and post-comparisons indicated a positive change both in the measurements collected by the therapists and also as described by Natalie herself. For example, Natalie's scores on the TAS showed a significant reduction in her score indicating that in this case alexithymia can be improved (Prince & Ford, 2012).

Goal 5: Natalie will learn to be compassionate to herself and develop a personal model of resilience

The Mood Week during the intensive phase took an integrated Compassion Focused and Cognitive Behavioural approach. Natalie also received weekly individual psychotherapy sessions and participated in a weekly support group with her peers, facilitated by two clinical psychologists.

Using Compassion Focused Therapy (CFT; Gilbert, 2005, 2010a, 2010b; Gilbert & Irons, 2005), Natalie and her psychologist developed a shared understanding of the psychological impact of the brain injury and how she coped with these challenges. Natalie felt criticised by others, often comparing herself unfavourably with them, leading to her feeling inadequate and threatened. She struggled to deal with the anxiety and anger these reactions triggered. She also struggled to calm or soothe herself when she had these feelings, which often led to her relying on others, as she did not feel able to comfort herself. Natalie's key goals for psychotherapy were 'to be as well as I can be in order to think about my future in terms of work, to not be ill each fortnight, to feel more energised and enthusiastic and less disconnected from others'. Natalie also wished to be able to cope better with the anxiety that she experienced in regard to her epilepsy. Psychotherapy sessions focused on learning and practising compassion focused techniques to increase self-soothing and reduce self-criticism as well as developing a personal model of resilience and learning to apply this to difficult situations.

As part of this work Natalie learnt Compassionate Mind Training (CMT) techniques, including soothing rhythm breathing and imagery exercises in the context of Compassion Focused Therapy and two-chair work. CMT helped Natalie to respond compassionately to herself in difficult situations. As part of this work, she developed a compassionate cue card to remind her to respond compassionately and ease her anxieties.

At the end of the programme, Natalie had made significant progress in managing the psychological challenges she faced as a result of the stroke.

She felt she was much better and thought she was doing what she wanted to do with her life. Questionnaire measures indicated that her anxiety had dropped to the borderline range, her depression symptoms had dropped to within the normal range, her self-esteem had risen to the normal range and her self-critical responses had also dropped, alongside an increase in her ability to reassure (soothe) herself. Given that Natalie had made such good progress, at the end of the programme it was recommended that she continue to see her psychologist monthly to ensure ongoing progress and to practise her relapse prevention plan, which she had recently completed.

During the programme, I got to concentrate on attention training techniques, as I needed to address attention issues as this could improve my memory. I also labelled my emotions and practised constructively expressing them as I was originally diagnosed with alexithymia. With my occupational therapist, we looked at work, as this was a big concern for the kind of things I could go on to do and whether I should consider going back to my old job as it was still an option for me. More importantly, we deciphered what really wasn't right for me, as I have a tendency to do what I think I 'should' do rather than what I want to do, especially when it comes to work!

In my Mood sessions with my psychologist I practised self-soothing and resilience strategies and have maintained a regular monthly session until recently. I was shown how to make use of a planning tool and encouraged to carry on making notes and putting everything in my diary, and my diary and post-it notes are now the two most sacred things on earth! With lots of persistence my new strategies have really helped me and made a big difference, and by the end of the programme my alexithymia scores were normal, which I was overjoyed about!

Goal 6: Natalie will explore her work skills and interest and develop a Work Identity Map

Natalie's main goal for these sessions with her occupational therapist was to explore her work skills and interests and develop a Work Identity Map by the end of the programme. She was on long-term sick leave from her job at the university. In order to understand the impact of the consequences of Natalie's stroke on this role, her OT developed a number of administrative tasks believed to reflect roles in her job for Natalie to complete at the centre under observation.

This assessment revealed a clear mismatch between the demands of the job and Natalie's skills and interests. Therefore, Natalie explored other areas of interest for work. For example, she ran an Art Group in the centre for both staff and clients. Natalie engaged well with this task and was given feedback on how to improve to make further achievements. Natalie was interested in setting up her own business drawing pet portraits. She independently initiated many of the tasks required to begin the process. She set up a project in the centre to trial this idea, and this proved to be a useful vehicle to explore the planning and pacing strategies she had been learning in order to overcome her cognitive difficulties and manage fatigue.

Natalie designed a task demands and environmental attributes list and found this to be useful and supportive in aiding her to return to work successfully. Examples from this included: having clear structure to her working day, with some flexibility to take into account fatigue and health requirements; limited time pressure, with more time to plan and perform certain tasks; having the opportunity to use creative skills and a clear outline of the task requirements and success criteria. This work was captured in a vocational identity map for Natalie to use and adapt as necessary. Natalie reported in the outcome meeting at the end of the programme that she had a much better idea of what work/vocation would suit her and what demands and attributes would be most helpful in future work. As compared to the start of the programme, ratings on the Canadian Occupation Performance Measure (COPM) (Law, Baptiste, McColl, Opzoomer, Polatajko & Pollock, 1990) indicated that her performance and satisfaction on functional areas had increased in all areas.

Goal 7: Natalie will produce an Understanding Brain Injury Project depicting her journey of recovery

As part of the integration phase, Natalie received 12 one-to-one UBI (Understanding Brain Injury) sessions focused on understanding how key areas (cognition, communication and emotions) were affected by her stroke. Part of this work involved accessing her medical records, including reports and notes to help her develop a timeline of events. She also viewed her MRI scans with support in interpreting their meaning as well as relating some of the areas to functional difficulties she experienced. Natalie chose to produce a piece of beautiful artwork in which she used the image of a phoenix to represent her recovery; this is depicted on the frontispiece of this book. Natalie also produced a poem to go with the picture to describe the journey:

As I rise from the ashes of my broken former self,
  I wonder where this torrid and unknown skyline is leading me?
  Uncertainly, I spread my wings and start to rise up,
  My wings start to gain momentum and I feel strong and free
again!
  In the distance I can see a small, white snowdrop.
  Its simplicity and purity is beautiful and draws me to it,
  Transmitting hope.

Outcome

Since leaving the programme, Natalie has continued her work as a pet portraitist, reporting that there is a slow but steady stream of customers and it is something that she enjoys. She also applied for and was successful in becoming an Ambassador for Service Users for the local mental health trust. This role is part time and involves increasing awareness of mental health problems and their impact from a service user's perspective. Natalie says she has found this role challenging but immensely satisfying. She feels better equipped to communicate how she is feeling with others in a helpful and assertive manner. She continues to use her strategies and feels she has significantly benefited from having longer-term psychotherapy to support her.

I find my role, as an Ambassador working with the trust, is valued. I hope, in its own small way I can make a positive difference to other people's lives who deserve and need it. It is wonderful to be doing something where I feel like my opinion is considered and listened to and where I hope we can make some positive changes for service users and their carers within the mental health system.

I still live with epilepsy, and life is far from easy at times due to anxiety about this, but I find strategies like the soothing breathing I was taught and having the Buddhist practice in my life gives me a lot of reassurance and comfort. I have started to use a technique called EFT (emotional freedom technique), which was introduced to me by my Buddhist friends and it helps me a lot too. I have also started a different type of Buddhist practice that was introduced to me by a friend, Maria, from an art studio I used to be a member of. I have noticed an inner contentment within myself since I have been practising this, and it is also wonderful to have the people that I have met through Buddhism in my life as well. Faith is a beautiful and powerful thing and it has given me a lot of strength but within a belief system that still allows me to feel free.

I've suffered quite a bit of depression and anxiety since having the spontaneous subarachnoid haemorrhage, which may have been due to changes in my brain chemistry, as a result of the damage to the right frontal lobe, or just the acceptance process I needed and am still going through. What I have found hugely helpful is time at the Buddhist centre, listening to music, talking to friends, going for walks or runs in the outdoors (when I'm feeling particularly energetic – nature is always amazing, and combining it with a bit of gentle exercise can be fantastic!) or the gym when it's too cold outside for that malarkey, the Oliver Zangwill team who have taught me SO very much about myself and my situation and that I'm not actually so bad after all! I feel I owe their expertise, care and kindness so very much and I will always be so incredibly grateful!

I also remind myself what my OT, Rachel, told me on my bad days, when I'm feeling down or exhausted and anxious about a seizure coming on I remember that I'm in a 10% survival rate with subarachnoid brain haemorrhages. This still gives me goose bumps and has a strong emotional reaction within me, making me think I must be here for a reason so I'm going to try and make this count!

For those in a similar position to me

Never think you are less of a person because this has happened to you. Life may be harder now for a while or for the foreseeable future but you will always be you. It may take some work to rediscover and get back to where you want to be and reconnect with all the precious individual talents that you have to offer, or it could be a case of discovering new ones, but what an adventure that will be!

For the health professionals

I think it's really important to really listen to the individual and be patient and give them enough time to think and talk and to say what they want to say as it can take longer and be harder to express what you're feeling and what you want to say after brain injury, and I've encountered this in a few different situations.

Chapter 4

Eliot's story
Rehabilitation through golf and family

Jill Winegardner and Eliot, Sue and David Ronaldson

Eliot was 19 years old when a terrible car crash left him with multiple fractures and a severe brain injury. After a good physical recovery, he tried school and work again but was not able to succeed because of cognitive difficulties, chiefly executive dysfunctions. With rehabilitation, he learned cognitive strategies, which, when combined with improved confidence and happiness as a result of programme successes, allowed him to move to his own cottage near his family. He has become a successful volunteer golf tutor for juniors and now hopes for paid employment.

Introduction

Eliot is the middle of three children in a close, supportive family from the East of England. He was an able student in school with good final examination results. His real passion, though, was golf and, after a gap year, he planned to take up a golf scholarship at an American university.

Background of injury

I was driving home from work in August 1997. I was a breakfast waiter at The Barns Hotel in Bedford, Bedfordshire as I was taking a year out, because in September 1997 I was going to Texas Wesleyan College in America on a golf scholarship.

The weather was perfect but at 11.30 am I drove off the road and went into a tree outside the Falcon Inn pub in Bledsoe, Bedfordshire. Fortunately, I had no passengers in the car because my front passenger seat ended up in the boot of the car. Due to the time of the accident and being close to the pub, two fire engines, two ambulances and a police car came to the site of the accident. My driver door had jammed so the fire service had to cut my car in two in order to get me out. The police went straight to my parents' house to explain what had happened. My mum grabbed the car keys but the police refused to let her drive as she would not be able to concentrate, so the police drove them to the hospital.

At Bedford Hospital Accident and Emergency they could not identify the problem to my head so they took me to Addenbrooke's Hospital in Cambridge. The journey normally takes around one hour but due to the machinery attached to me, the journey took three hours.

When they are sent to hospital most people are scared, but for me Addenbrooke's was heaven, it is incredible what they can do. In hospital I had a CT scan, which showed I had left side bruising to my brain so I was placed in an induced coma. I had fractured my skull bone, pelvis, cheek bone and right arm. Due to the fact that I deteriorated on the eighth day, Rodney Laing, my surgeon, decided to remove part of my skull, which took place on 6 September 1997. A plate was inserted, then my skull was replaced on 29 October 1997. As well as my skull, my arm was opened and a pin inserted, and a plate was inserted into my cheek bone to the fractures. All the operations had to be done, for which I am very thankful.

Being in hospital for so long, I became very isolated and quiet. On leaving hospital nothing could have been better than communication with friends and family.

The support of Eliot's family was crucial in his recovery. We asked his parents, Sue and David, to share their story with us.

In August 1997, on a bright, sunny morning, our witty, intelligent, loving son hit a tree while driving home from work, resulting in him suffering a severe head injury, fractures to his facial bones and forearm and a collapsed lung, which unbeknown to us at the time was to change his life, our life and the lives of his sisters forever.

The cause of the crash was never established as there were no signs of excessive speed and no other vehicle was involved. A possible cause was that Eliot had fainted at the wheel as he had made no attempt at braking.

Eliot was rushed to Bedford Hospital where he was given initial life-saving treatment and put on a ventilator. After the first brain scan a decision was made to transfer him to the Neurological Critical Care Unit at Addenbrooke's Hospital. During the first week, Eliot's brain swelling fluctuated dramatically and he was maintained on full life support. The swelling increased so much and so rapidly at the end of the week that an emergency craniectomy had to be performed to save his life. Our lives were in turmoil.

During the following week Eliot's brain swelling decreased and surgery to his fractured jaw and forearm and a tracheostomy were performed. It was then decided to wean him off the ventilator, and it was with absolute relief and joy when Eliot finally opened his eyes and smiled and appeared to recognise us all. He could hear us and see us, and when a ball was gently thrown at him he caught it single-handedly. His hand-to-eye coordination appeared to be intact. However, over the following days, came the painful realisation that Eliot's memory had been severely impaired. He could not remember his name, where he lived, where he was or why he was in hospital.

His PTA [post-traumatic amnesia] lasted for many worrying weeks and for this reason his transfer to the Rehabilitation Unit was postponed. Transfer was finally made after his skull had been replaced. During his time in rehabilitation his progress was painfully slow. All he wanted to do was pretend to swing a golf club and talk about golf. He became very agitated at times and it was very upsetting to watch. You felt so helpless.

Eliot: *The worry they must have been through with the position I was in is incredible. The relief that must have been felt on my release from hospital is incredible. For me it has shown that nothing can beat your family. One thing is, is that I could never forget both the love that they have given me and the love that I have for them.*

Sue and David: *As Eliot wasn't suffering from any physical problems such as epileptic seizures etc., we persuaded the doctors to let us take him home where we hoped his progress might be better in his own home with his familiar things around him. We could take him to the golf club where he could play the game he loved, and could still play to a high standard amongst friends he knew. This he did with the watchful eye of the Club Pro and other members of the club who were so supportive.*

He gradually grew stronger physically and although his short-term memory remained very poor, also his problem solving, he began to do more and more independently, although needing constant reminders.

Eliot: *One area of therapy that I decided to take was to join Headway, which is a national service set up to rehabilitate people with head problems. The first months of sessions that I used the facility ran well, but in time the service became uninteresting because the majority of time was spent just sitting down speaking to people while drinking tea or coffee, instead of actually covering any skills that could have an influence on the damage that had been caused to my brain.*

From spending the majority of time staying at home at my parents' house I decided that I had to do something to both get out of the house and use my brain. From going to hospital I could appreciate that I had a brain due to the fact that it expanded in the accident.

My first attempt was to go into Bedford and do an NVQ on computing. This was very beneficial because I was able to achieve NVQ Level III, which is useful for many jobs and I was also able to communicate with other students.

A few years on, I went and studied a course on Golf Course Management. This course was based at Merrist Wood College in Surrey. The course gave me the opportunity to study and communicate with other students and to have more independence in the way I lived. Unfortunately, I was unable to receive a qualification but it gave me the drive and ambition for the future.

January 14 2004 was a day that considerably changed my life. I am associated with a society called Papworth, and on this day they gave me a flat in Bedford. The flat was based just out of the town but it was easy access into town. The best results of moving into the flat were the independence it gave me and also the responsibility to maintain my own accommodation, but also the responsibility to look after my bills for essentials and food.

Sue and David: We did, however, struggle to find the professional assistance that he so badly needed. He did attend Headway but just got bored with painting and basket making! He was an 18-year-old who loved sport and the outdoors and was missing his friends who had all moved on to universities, where they were getting on with their lives.

Life can be extremely cruel.

We were referred by our doctor to the Acquired Brain Injury Services in Dunstable where Eliot attended an assessment, and consequently received a few half-hourly sessions with a neuropsychologist. During this time he successfully completed an NVQ in computing and then decided to attempt the Business Studies Course at Westminster University in London that he had been accepted for before his accident. However, it soon became all too clear that he could not cope with this and he subsequently returned home.

He did then manage to acquire a Papworth Trust flat in Bedford and he began to live independently. He also attended a comprehensive Driving Assessment at the Nuffield Orthopaedic Centre in Oxford and passed successfully, which did boost his confidence and morale. He then managed to find work in retail for two or three years but lost his job and then began to get progressively more and more depressed. Out of work, living on his own and seemingly unable to make new friends, he became unable to cope financially, began drinking more, became more aggressive and at times felt suicidal.

Eliot was already 12 years post-injury and his family was desperate to find help for him. Eliot wanted a 'normal life' with work and a family of his own. His sisters and schoolmates were getting married and starting families while he felt left out of these major life milestones. This made him sad and lonely. His parents felt that Eliot was consuming too much beer, especially when he was depressed. At these times, he became irritable and angry with his family.

Eliot: *My elder sister fortunately found the Oliver Zangwill Centre (OZC) on the internet. This gave a promising aspect to my rehabilitation due to the fact that no other centre had been of any benefit.*

Sue and David: *At this time we were desperate for help for him. A friend's daughter who happened to be an occupational therapist at The National Hospital in London put us in touch with the Oliver Zangwill Centre, but of course there was the matter of funding to be considered. Eliot's doctor wrote to the PCT [Primary Care Trust, the funding body for the National Health Service], who would only consider funding if an initial assessment was made by the Acquired Head Injury Unit in Dunstable. This was duly done but they did not recommend Eliot to be a suitable candidate for OZC as they felt he was not engaging with them. But, as an assessment at OZC pointed out, that was because he had a head injury! The PCT would not therefore provide any funding.*

We as a family were not satisfied with this and were determined to do everything we could to acquire a place for Eliot at OZC. An initial assessment was made and it was felt that Eliot would benefit from the professional expertise of the team at OZC.

Assessment

Eliot and his parents came for a two-day assessment to identify his rehabilitation needs in detail (see Chapter 1). He was a pleasant, friendly young man with an indentation in his forehead due to surgical repair following his injury, but no other physical signs of injury. He interacted well with staff and even volunteered to present a news item at the daily community meeting. His speech was quick and sometimes unintelligible. Eliot answered questions with short responses and asked few questions. He tended to talk about a small range of topics and sometimes got 'stuck' on a topic rather than flexibly moving to a new idea. His range of emotional expression was appropriate to the content of conversations though somewhat blunted.

Eliot showed superficial awareness of deficits. He was fully aware of the emotional consequences of his situation, expressing feelings of depression and loneliness at the lack of friends and social life, and anxiety over having no work. He could verbalise brain-injury related deficits such as irritability and memory loss but, when pressed, acknowledged that he knew about these things because others had told him so, rather than through personal awareness and understanding of them. His lack of acknowledgement of his deficits appeared to be due to a true inability to recognise them rather than resistance or psychological denial as, when they were pointed out, he agreed and could see the problem. He simply could not make the connections between his life problems and his brain-injury related impairments (Prigatano, 2005). Eliot reported physical changes, including diminished sense of smell and taste and occasional sleep disturbance. Mild fatigue was noted by his parents but not recognised by Eliot. There were no other physical problems.

Eliot's main cognitive challenges were with aspects of attention and memory and, most important, we identified executive difficulties as being at the heart of Eliot's problems. These included concreteness, problems with initiative and carry through of plans, difficulty monitoring and reflecting on thoughts and actions consistently and trouble generating and elaborating thoughts and ideas. These executive difficulties showed up on cognitive testing, during the community outing and on the functional task, as well as in informal observations when Eliot navigated his way around the centre. Eliot clearly benefited from structure and routine on tests, per community observations, and per his parents' report, doing well when structure was provided. We created an interdisciplinary formulation of Eliot's executive functioning (see Figure 4.1).

Eliot talked about the difficulties with mood and relationships he had experienced since his head injury. He said that he was slightly more irritable and aggressive in conversation, which affected his family relationships. His triggers included perceived criticism from others or his own sense of not doing something well. He described getting 'wound up' faster and more intensely than before his accident and responding by becoming louder and snappy. He even once hit his head against the wall in frustration. After outbursts he calms fairly quickly and feels annoyed and embarrassed about them. He attributes outbursts to not thinking before acting. Eliot had no strategies to manage his anger when he first came to us.

Eliot reported considerable loneliness since losing touch with friends following his accident. He lived alone and had no close friends although he socialised with acquaintances several times a week. He found this boring and un-motivating and sometimes put off tasks because there was no one else with him. He felt very low on a daily basis unless he was doing something, such as shopping, playing golf or being with people. However, he had little money to spend, as he was not working. Lack of work was also a source of worries. His scores on the Hospital Anxiety and Depression Scale (HADS) (Zigmond & Snaith, 1983) indicated borderline levels of both anxiety and depression.

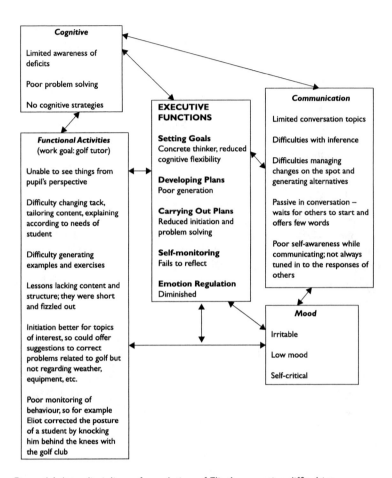

Figure 4.1 Interdisciplinary formulation of Eliot's executive difficulties.

Eliot: *The problem was, the PCT of Bedford were not going to pay for the service. This meant that we had to raise £30,000 in order to be treated at the centre. Fortunately family and friends began schemes in order to raise the money. Ross, my younger brother-in-law, competed with friends in a British Triathlon competition and all money from sponsorship was kindly received, and Richard, my older brother-in-law, competed with a colleague of his in a half Iron Man competition and thankfully raised a great value for my rehabilitation.*

Sue and David: *Again, the issue of funding had to be overcome. Not to be daunted, our two wonderful sons-in-law took on the challenge. One completed the Bedford*

Triathlon and the other the Texas Half Iron Man and between them raised the magnificent sum of over £30,000. We can never thank them and all who sponsored them enough. Eliot could finally get the help he so desperately needed.

Rehabilitation

Thanks to his family, Eliot was now ready to start the intensive rehabilitation programme. Rehabilitation goals were generated based on the formulation from the assessment and the problem list generated by Eliot and his family.

Goal 1: Improve awareness

This goal was addressed in the intensive phase. Eliot and the other three clients in his group learned about the key topics of brain function, attention and memory, executive functions, communication and mood through multimedia presentations, exercises, quizzes, reflecting on their own experiences, trying out strategies for managing related problems and putting their strategies into practice through activities in the Centre (Fleming & Ownsworth, 2006).

Goal 2: Use strategies

Work on this goal began in the group phase and continued in individual cognitive sessions. Eliot learned and tried out various strategies to help manage his cognitive difficulties. For example, he was taught the Goal Management Framework (GMF). Based on the work of Duncan (1986) and Robertson (1996), the GMF is a six-step problem-solving strategy:

1   What is my goal?
2   What are my options to reach the goal?
3   List pros and cons of each option and make a choice.
4   Plan the steps.
5   Do it! Carry out the plan.
6   Reflect, adjust, evaluate.

The GMF process helped Eliot stay focused on his goal and helped him 'think outside the box' with its emphasis on generating several options for each plan. He learned to attend to the process of generating ideas by taking part in behavioural experiments where he was first asked to predict how many ideas he could generate and then asked to generate ideas. For example, he was asked to predict how many ideas he could generate for Christmas gifts for his family, and then he generated ideas before reflecting on his prediction. He soon found himself generating far more ideas than he predicted just by focusing his attention on the task.

Another tool that helped Eliot think more diversely was 'Stop–Think'. This simple concept was introduced to encourage Eliot to reflect on his thoughts, evaluate them, and monitor them more closely. He added a variant, which was 'Stop–Think Do I Have Enough?' He wrote this phrase on the first page of his Filofax, as well as at home and on his golf bag, and was prompted to use it in a variety of situations.

Eliot looked at memory and planning tools, and he decided on a small Filofax with sections for a calendar, things-to-do list and notes. He used the calendar to keep track of appointments and to review the day, and he referred to his things-to-do list routinely and ticked off completed items. Eliot carried the Filofax at all times and referred to it frequently until it became an automatic habit.

Goal 3: Volunteer/work interests and planning

Progress towards the third goal was guided by Eliot's occupational therapist (OT). One of his interests was cooking, and he chose to cook lunch for the staff. He used the GMF with his OT's support to choose a menu, plan the required steps and carry out the task. He selected an appropriate stir fry recipe, bought the correct ingredients in the right quantities and set the table up nicely. However, there was not enough food to go around and staff members either had very small portions or had to go to the cafeteria! Later, in reflecting with his OT, Eliot identified the problem as the fact that the wok was too small to hold all the ingredients he had purchased, so he only cooked enough food to fit in the wok. Although he did not use the GMF to solve the problem at the time, with his OT's support, he was later able to generate several alternative solutions that would have saved the day.

His OT realised that Eliot needed a good deal of pre-planning and structure to be successful. As he wanted to be a golf tutor, she thought about the ways his executive functioning difficulties might impact on success. The two of them hatched a plan for Eliot to offer golf lessons to the staff and clients during lunch breaks. He was videotaped during the lessons and each student completed a feedback form. From this information, the OT identified ways that executive difficulties impacted on Eliot's tutoring ability, as described in Figure 4.1.

Eliot showed both strengths and challenges during his golf lessons. He kept focused on the task and was not distracted, and showed good initiation. He circulated fliers to clients and staff, put a 'sign up' list in the common room and chased staff and clients for commitment to lessons.

His OT developed several strategies to help Eliot overcome his executive difficulties. She taught him to use short phrases and mnemonics to structure the session and think about whether he had enough content. She helped him expand his repertoire by developing his ability to ask himself the four Ws and an H (what, why, when, where, how) and to think about three key tutor behaviours: demonstrate, observe and reflect. She utilised Eliot's golf knowledge by encouraging him to use analogies he had learned in the past to explain things to students. Together, they gathered a library of exercises for Eliot to have at hand.

Next, they set up a structure for the lessons and wrote a plan for what went into each – beginning, middle and end. At first, the OT guided Eliot through this process and later encouraged him to fill out a pro forma. Although he was able to do this, he needed prompting for extra detail. He continued to use his GMF strategy to make decisions. They then laminated the lesson plan sheets so that Eliot could use them repeatedly.

After Eliot had practised his new skills by giving lessons to a fellow client, his OT set up a volunteer work placement for him with his local golf club. The placement included shadowing the golf professional and then teaching under supervision, using his own eight-week set of lesson plans. Throughout his placement, his OT helped Eliot reflect on his performance and use feedback to improve it. She gave clear and explicit ground rules regarding behaviour, such as no drinking at the club or asking women golfers for dates. Eliot used his 'Stop–Think' strategy to reflect on the suitability of his comments and behaviour at the golf course with good success.

Goal 4: Social communication

The fourth goal focused on helping Eliot to improve his conversational skills and to increase his social participation. His speech and language therapist (SALT) listed the ways Eliot's executive functioning difficulties hindered him socially (as seen in Figure 4.1). She observed that his difficulties in generating ideas resulted in a limited number of conversation topics. Concrete thinking made it hard for Eliot to interpret inference. Reduced flexibility of thinking meant that Eliot had trouble managing changes on the spot, and in thinking of alternatives. Low initiation meant that he was passive in conversations, usually waiting for others to start them. Reduced self-monitoring resulted in Eliot some-times being unaware of the impact of his own behaviour (verbal and non-verbal) and others' responses.

The SALT worked with the OT to observe Eliot during his golf lessons. She videotaped the classes to observe Eliot's communication and speech, noticing that he tended to speak too rapidly and had trouble organising his comments in a logical sequence. She regarded Eliot's confidence with the topic of golf and his enthusiasm as a teacher as real strengths.

His SALT helped Eliot improve his verbal communication skills in preparation for a professional role by reviewing the videos with him, using a golfing DVD as a model, and encouraging him to practise communication skills by chairing community meetings, presenting news items to the team and giving another series of golf lessons to a fellow client. In all of these activities, his SALT supported him in practising self-monitoring and focusing on non-verbal skills such as increasing his eye contact.

Another goal that Eliot set with his SALT was to develop social confidence through exploring social opportunities. They decided to use a speed-dating event as a vehicle for Eliot to plan and prepare for social opportunities. The SALT worked together with Eliot's cognitive therapist to create a GMF for speed dating. With their help, Eliot planned all the details, including travelling to and from the event and purchasing tickets, as well as generating conversation starters and topics and thinking about what to wear. These activities involved setting goals, planning and organising the details, problem solving and generating ideas. Eliot practised conversation skills with his SALT in individual sessions and then she organised a practice event with volunteers from the staff. She sat the volunteers at tables around the room and had a timer telling Eliot when to move from table to table. Eliot did very well with all of the preparation for the speed dating, including the practice event. Unfortunately, when he was meant to book his place, he was asked for bank details and did not wish to give them. He was unable to problem solve an alternative and lost his place on the night. The learning outcome was to focus even more on 'Stop–Think' and problem-solving skills with Eliot.

Goal 5: Psychological support

This goal was pursued through the provision of individual psycho-therapy. Eliot learned strategies to manage his irritability though his family said his irritability vanished once he started the programme.

Eliot's psychotherapy then focused on maintaining his confidence and increasing his participation in enjoyable activities.

Goal 6: Family education and support

The sixth goal was tackled by inviting Eliot's family to educational days at the OZC, family groups for families of clients, and individual progress and review meetings with Eliot. Eliot's programme coordinator regularly phoned his mother to see how he was progressing, to update her on rehabilitation activities and to answer questions. Family feedback was incorporated into rehab planning throughout the programme. Eliot was fortunate to have such a strong and supportive family throughout his rehabilitation, and this was a key factor in his success (Oddy & Herbert, 2003).

We determined the success of the programme through the achievement of the goals set. Eliot achieved all of his goals and his rehabilitation was considered to be successful. We believe that we had helped him through a combination of a) using his existing skills more efficiently, and b) finding other routes to attain his targets through the use of compensatory strategies. It is also possible that, to some extent, we were restoring lost function.

Today, Eliot has moved to a cottage near his family where he lives independently. He successfully continues to volunteer teaching golf to juniors and he and his family report his mood is good and his irritability has vanished. Nevertheless, he has not yet been able to find paid work. He came back to the OZC for some booster sessions to work on his CV and job-seeking skills, but the poor economy and some geographical restrictions have prevented this goal to date. He is now linked in with local brain injury services and participates in a job-seeking group. We believe that Eliot will be successful in paid work once the hurdle of finding the right job has been overcome.

Eliot: *On joining the OZC I was very nervous and worried about the people I was going to be with and what the actual process was going to be. Hence progressing with the rehabilitation has changed my life. Due to the great support from the staff and meeting some new friends I have now learnt some new strategies (especially 'Stop–Think' and the use of GMF. I have now become much more confident with communication with my family and have the drive to advance in life.*

Sue and David: *Eliot attended the 18-week course and to our amazement his demeanour changed quite quickly as he began to understand the complexities of* the injury he sustained and how to learn new coping strategies. He became less agitated, aggressive and despondent. At last he and we felt that he was being understood and specifically and generally helped to cope with, and overcome, some of the difficulties he faces.

OZC has also very much helped us as a family to help him in the best way possible. We understand that his injuries were so severe that he will always face difficulties and we have had to come to terms with the fact that the light-hearted, witty son we once knew has changed in so many ways, but for us learning to cope with him in testing times has helped enormously. To know that OZC and all the wonderful professionals who have helped us will always be there for us has brought huge relief to us all.

We cannot thank you all enough and long may you continue the magnificent work you do in helping all those who have had the misfortune to have had their lives so cruelly changed forever; you have given them hope for the future.

Chapter 5

Kate's story
Recovery takes time, so don't give up

Barbara A. Wilson and Kate Bainbridge

Kate, a teacher living with her boyfriend, became ill with a form of encephalitis. She was in a state of low responsiveness for several months. Although severely physically handicapped, she has continued to improve for 14 years. She engages fully in life and is a true heroine. We wrote about Kate in Wilson et al. *(2009). This chapter is an update on Kate's progress since then.*

Introduction

Kate was born in 1970, the second daughter of a professional family living in Cambridge. She had a happy normal childhood with no serious illnesses. Her older sister trained as a medical doctor and Kate went to university to study history. After completing her degree Kate trained as a primary school teacher. In 1997 she was living with her boyfriend and her life was full and happy.

Background of illness

Shortly before her 27th birthday, Kate developed a sore throat and a headache. Her mother described what happened.

Mrs Bainbridge: *One Sunday Kate phoned to say she had a sore throat. On Monday she went to work. I phoned on Tuesday but didn't speak to Kate, I spoke to Kate's boyfriend. He said Kate was not well and was in bed. He went to work on Wednesday and when he came home he could not wake her. He telephoned an ambulance and Kate was taken to hospital where she was said to be in a coma. They didn't know what was wrong. The next day a doctor came from Addenbrooke's and said Kate had to go straight there. He had arranged the ambulance. I was relieved as he was a neighbour of ours so was known to us. She went to Addenbrooke's where it was difficult for them to diagnose her condition but she was found to have an acute disseminated encephalomyelopathy. Dr A said that although they knew it was encephalitis they could not identify the particular virus. He also said that Kate's immune system had not switched off so we took that to mean that Kate had damage from the encephalitis together with damage from the immune system attacking the brainstem.*

A CT scan at the time showed diffuse cerebral swelling with a large ventroponto medullary (brainstem) lesion and lesions in both thalami. An MRI scan confirmed this. Kate was found to have damage in the brainstem, to both thalami and both medial temporal lobes.

At that time Kate was not responding to commands, she showed no consistent spontaneous or elicited motor responses or eye movements and she was not able to communicate. She had a sleep–wake cycle, however, and anecdotal evidence suggested that she occasionally followed family members with her eyes. It was concluded she was in a vegetative state.

Kate regained some awareness 5–6 months after the onset of her illness. In May 1998, that is 11 months after onset, she was admitted to a rehabilitation centre where she spent a further 11 months.

In June 1997 I got an odd form of ADEM encephalitis, only my mid brainstem was attacked. My memory and mind were untouched so I had normal intellectual functioning. Even so, I had rather a lot to come to terms with, deal with and cope with and my life had changed rather a lot. I can't walk or even sit up on my own. I have just started talking but I can't eat or drink.

I went into a coma and remained unconscious for about four months. Then slowly I became conscious, but it took a few months to be conscious all day. My recovery has been very slow; so far it has been continuing for almost 15 years.

In April 1999 Kate was discharged home under the care of her parents, where she lived until December 2008. Every few weeks she spent two weeks in respite care. It was while she was there that the request was received to assess her cognitive abilities.

Assessment

I spent 22 months in hospital, which was not fun at all. I was treated like a body, not a person with feelings or someone having full mental skills. I can remember the psychologist coming to my bed in hospital. I didn't know who he was and

I couldn't hear him. At that time words were just noise to me. So I was rather scared from that meeting; they said I was untestable. People should be tested every few months, as in recovery people change. I found it took about two years for my brain to cope with the huge shock of the effects of my illness.

The first assessment lasted for three hours spread over two visits. I went to the respite home one afternoon, not quite sure what tests to take or how interactive Kate would be. She was in a wheelchair and used a letter board to communicate because of severe dysarthria. I explained to Kate that I wanted to assess her understanding, thinking, memory and concentration. I opened the Raven's Standard Progressive Matrices (a non-verbal test of reasoning) and explained to her about the test. Very quickly she became engrossed in the task and worked out many of the solutions. I realised that Kate was less impaired than I had expected and I had taken the wrong tests with me, so I said I would come again in a few days with more tests. The next time Kate managed to complete a number of tests either through pointing to the correct answer/response or through spelling out the answers on her letter board.

Kate was assessed with tests of reasoning, verbal intelligence and memory. My conclusions at the end of the assessment were that Kate was probably functioning a little below her previous level of ability. However, almost none of the results were in the impaired range. At the very least she was functioning in the low average range, and for someone who had been vegetative/minimally conscious for several months this was excellent. Kate was feeling distressed when first seen and this could have depressed her scores. She also had relatively poor vision so that material needed to be close to her or in large print for her to see it well.

In August and September 2000, Kate was reassessed. Her mood at this time was much better. She could discuss what had happened to her without becoming distressed and spelled out on her letter board that she enjoyed doing the tests as it showed people she was not stupid. She had improved on most of the tests and was in the average range or above, apart from recognition memory for faces. This had improved but was still below the fifth percentile. Additional tests were given to Kate over the following year. She did consistently well and tests showed her problem-solving ability and her capacity to 'keep on track' were good.

After the assessment in September 2000, Kate asked me for a letter to summarise the results. I wrote the following communication that Kate kept for many years.

To whom it may concern

Kate Bainbridge was taken ill with an infection of the brain in 1997. For about six months she remained in a minimally conscious state. This means she was able to open her eyes and showed a sleep–wake cycle but could not communicate, respond to situations or show evidence of thinking. Since that time Kate has made considerable progress, indeed she is fairly unusual in showing such good recovery in her thinking and memory. People who are so severely impaired for so long rarely achieve the level Kate has attained. She is to be congratulated for achieving so much.

Although Kate is severely disabled physically and has difficulty with her speech, her thinking and reasoning skills are within the normal range. It is easy for people to underestimate her intelligence given her speech and motor problems. This is likely to prove frustrating for Kate and may well make her angry.

For someone in Kate's position, it is important to have consistency in her life and for her to be cared for by people she can trust and who understand her problems. Anybody who has sustained an injury to the brain is likely to weep more readily, to become fatigued more easily and to find certain situations frustrating. Given Kate's dependence on others for physical care and her need to communicate with her board, these tendencies are likely to be exacerbated. She will probably respond best to understanding and approval rather than criticism.

In many ways Kate is a remarkable young woman, given how far she has come since those first six months after her illness, and she needs opportunities to show her intellectual capacities.

The best thing in my recovery that made me try and keep going was being assessed by Barbara Wilson. This happened about six weeks after I left hospital. When I was in hospital my mum asked if I could see Barbara as she had heard about her from the Encephalitis Society, but was told I couldn't see her. Anyway, I was glad as I was so scared and worried in hospital.

Barbara's tests made my brain come alive. Before her tests I had questions in my mind but I was not able to take part in the world. Her tests set my mind free. I also found out that Barbara likes cats and I love them too.

Barbara made me want to say jokes. In her first test I thought of a joke but I didn't dare say it as I thought I had to be serious. She asked me who was the

President of the USA; it was the time of Clinton and his affair so I wanted to say Monica Lewinsky!

Her tests also gave me confidence. She said I had average scores on my tests; that was so good to hear. I knew I was fine, I just needed someone to agree with me! My parents knew I was fine in that area, but Barbara's test results were proof that could not be argued with.

Kate was certainly appreciative of the assessments and the letter. She was very angry at her treatment in hospital. When I first knew her she frequently expressed her anger. Her parents discussed this with me and it soon became a focus of our treatment. In October 2000, Kate sent me a letter saying,

Thank you so much for the assessments. They treated me as if I was stupid (in hospital). My stay there was absolute hell, they never told me anything. They used to suction me through my mouth and they never told me why, or what it was called, they have never told me about my trachy (tracheostomy tube). I am lucky I am with it and have a good memory so I could work it out. I don't want them to do it to anyone else. They have learnt a lot from me already, but I think telling people what you are doing is very important. I can't tell you how frightening it was, especially suction through the mouth. I tried to hold my breath to get away from all the pain. They never told me about my (feeding) tube. I wondered why I did not eat.

Early in January 2001, I received another letter from Kate saying,

Thank you so much for the letter about me, it will really help. I knew I was OK, my memory has been fine since the end of October 1997. I can remember the physio asking me why I made so much noise. Well, I was screaming as they caused me so much pain. I don't want anybody to have the same awful time as I did. I think my case shows you don't treat people as textbook cases. You need to be told where you are every day for a few months and make sure they can hear you. It sounded just like noise to me, even though my hearing tests showed no hearing loss. It is really frightening not knowing where I was or why I was there. No doctor ever told me about my illness. They are lucky I am with it, I worked it all out.

Kate, Fergus Gracey, a trainee with me at the time, and I wrote a paper about Kate's cognitive recovery (Wilson, Gracey & Bainbridge, 2001).

Kate said to me in 2007 that she was treated as a body and not a person: she felt there was no hope for her. Her mother said that everyone was very kind in the first hospital but did not know what was wrong. In the second hospital in intensive care her parents were told they could ring any time day or night so they felt involved. After about four or five weeks Kate was moved to the specialist head injury ward and although the staff were always willing to talk, and were honest, there was no sense of excitement.

Mrs Bainbridge: *When I told them that Kate moved her fingers today they said 'not to read too much into that as babies move their fingers'. I felt distressed about that. Once I got angry with them and said they shouldn't talk about Kate as if she wasn't there. She had speech and OT and we were trying to communicate. She had no facial expression. We tried blinking and couldn't get that right. Then we used a Yes/No board and then her sister came and brought a big pad with felt tip pens and we wrote things like, 'We love you'. We discovered she hated TV. We'd put it on when we left thinking it would provide some company but she hated it. Kate said at this point, 'I couldn't hear it'.*

For a long time Kate heard noises but could not understand speech.

Mrs Bainbridge: *I would wheel her round the hospital, holding Kate's head up with one hand and pushing the wheelchair with the other. Sometimes we would be crying.*

Kate's father said that on one occasion he told one of the staff that he was thinking of buying a computer for Kate and was told that there wasn't much point. The computer now, of course, is crucially important for Kate. In contrast, one of the senior nurses there said to Kate's parents, 'Never give up', and when Kate went to rehabilitation they had a very good social worker for a time so it was not all bad. Indeed, the family feel they had some good treatment but so many things were not dealt with well. They have certainly had to battle to move forwards.

When I left hospital 22 months after I became ill, we were told that any more recovery was unlikely and I would probably stay as I was. I could make hardly any noise nor could I move much. I now talk and do not use the letter board and I have just moved to a bungalow with a live-in carer as I have a tracheostomy (not for breathing but because I can't clear my lungs). So you can't put any time limit on recovery. When I was first ill they said most recovery was in the first six weeks! Six years is very quick for me!

I think they assumed many things as I had encephalitis, but I was an odd case.

Rehabilitation

The management of emotional difficulties is an essential part of neuropsychological rehabilitation (Prigatano, 1999). Without such treatment we are likely to reduce the chances of successful rehabilitation. Between 2000 and 2007, Kate was seen by several clinical psychology trainees, each of whom were spending a few months with me as part of their training (Macniven et al., 2003).

During her first few months in hospital Kate had several chest infections and reduced muscle power. Consequently, the main focus for this period of rehabilitation was physiotherapy, which, as we saw earlier, Kate found frightening and painful. Behavioural difficulties, including screaming and occasional biting, were recorded but no one offered help with her cognitive, emotional and behavioural problems.

Once the cognitive assessment had been carried out and it was clear that Kate was functioning better than expected by many of those working with her, we realised that we should try to help her deal with the emotional problems. Kate's psychological reaction to her illness was considerable. Premorbidly, Kate was reported by her family to have been very bright, kind, shy and quiet. She had achieved a good first degree, followed by a post-graduate teaching qualification. Kate was in a long-term relationship with her boyfriend. They had just bought a house together and had plans to marry. Her parents and family were close. Following her illness, Kate's relationships, employment, social existence and identity had all altered. At a stage when she had been thinking about marriage and a family, her illness appeared to have changed everything. Not surprisingly, Kate experienced low mood, anger and anxiety reactions, which reflected the shocking change in her circumstances.

During her time in rehabilitation and while on respite, Kate presented as withdrawn and depressed. She was prone to screaming, especially during physiotherapy, and was known to bite other people – often this would be when others would be helping with her personal care. Kate's behaviour could be seen as an attempt to communicate to those providing her care that she was frightened and in pain. Kate's difficulties with communication and her reliance upon a communication board often resulted in frustration for her and her carers, as misunderstandings would be common.

Since her original treatment in hospital, Kate had begun to feel very angry about the way she felt she had been treated. This became a dominant theme in her discussion of what had happened to her, persisting for a number of years. This anger and frustration that Kate felt was also at times directed towards her family and friends and towards herself:

I have just met an old friend from uni and it really upset me. I can now see how much I am missing. She has been married for five years and she has a house and a life. I just scream as I can't cry, which I would do if I could. I hate feeling guilty. I was carefree before and now I rely on others.

From a cognitive-behavioural perspective, Kate's depression could be seen to involve suicidal ideation, a sense of worthlessness and a pattern of negative thinking, feeling, behaviour and physical sensation. It was clear that Kate's insight into the changes in her life was increasing and with it the realisation that she had lost a great deal. The enormous task of beginning to recognise the changes in her life now and in the future was beginning to become clear to Kate at the point at which she began therapy. Kate reflected:

I feel depressed as it will be ages before I can get married. If I ever can ... I also know that I will never be well enough to have a baby, which is very hard to cope with as I used to want lots ... I also feel guilty as I know I am hard work.

Formulation

In formulating the psychological distress that Kate was experiencing, we considered that the environmental factors such as her continued inter-action problems with carers, and internal factors such as her pattern of negative thinking and behavioural avoidance, were keeping Kate focused on the past and on what she had lost. It was as if Kate was stuck in the trauma she had experienced and was overwhelmed with this loss of normality. Kate's self-esteem was low, now describing herself as 'stupid' and 'useless'. Formulation allowed for specific patterns of thinking and behaviour to be explored with Kate.

I had more tests over the next few years and really enjoyed them. Barbara also saw I had a lot of anger due to the results of my illness and my experiences. She gave me neuropsychology. That was so good, I can't say how much it has helped me and made me think about what had happened to me. I had been hoping since I got ill that I would get back to how I was before and everything would be a bad dream, but now I can see it is for real and I need to make a new life.

The most important thing was neuropsychology made me realise what had happened and made me think. It helped me to get my anger under control and it made me understand what had happened to me. I think neuropsychology should be used more, as after such a shock as brain injury you need help to make a new life and come to terms with what has happened, no matter how much or how little your mental skills have been affected. You need to realise this is life now and you need to make it a happy life. I had neuropsychology for a few years. Like everything else, you can't put a time limit on it. I can't say how much it helped me cope with everything and see that the effects of this illness just won't go away. So meeting Barbara, being assessed properly, and having help in dealing with my anger helped my recovery and helped me to cope.

The main purposes of our intervention were to reduce Kate's distress and anger and to help her understand herself better. A key element of effective psychotherapy is the development of a therapeutic alliance.

Many individuals who experience brain injury do not have the opportunity to benefit from psychotherapy as part of their rehabilitation. Some people believe that brain injury is a legitimate reason for excluding someone from psychotherapy, and that cognitive problems may prevent 'carryover' from session to session. We disagree, and would argue that the heterogeneous nature of brain injury is a good reason why a psychological formulation should be incorporated into an individual's comprehensive rehabilitation. By developing a detailed understanding of the individual's situation from the person's perspective, a tailored approach to therapy, drawing on multiple theoretical perspectives, can be undertaken. The work with Kate involved elements and techniques from a number of theoretical perspectives in an attempt to draw upon the strengths of each as they applied to Kate and her situation.

A variety of treatment approaches including personal construct theory, anger management techniques, cognitive behaviour therapy and mindfulness training enabled Kate to focus more on the present, to think realistically and optimistically about her future, and to interact more successfully with carers. Kate reported in 2006:

I can't believe how much I have changed. I now want to be alive and I am looking forward to the future ... I can now keep myself occupied and busy, instead of sitting on my own doing nothing ... I just don't want anyone else to have such an awful time as me, I can now see it is over and hopefully I will never have it again ... Can you see how angry I used to feel? But now there is no point in being angry, I just need to look to the future.

Kate's family was enormously influential in her emotional recovery and gave Kate the chance to adjust. Without this support it is unlikely that Kate could have recovered to the extent that she has. In fact, it is certain that this was the most important protective factor that prevented Kate from having a much worse experience, and contributed very significantly to Kate's cognitive and emotional recovery. It is vital that families are given the support they themselves need in order that they can positively influence the outcome of the person who has sustained a brain injury (Tyerman & Booth, 2001). As Kate says:

I am very lucky to have my Mum and Dad. I just feel so sorry for people who don't have my Mum and Dad, they will be on their own in hospital with no one to look after them. I am just glad I had Mum, Dad and my boyfriend to be my friends: they do so much for me and keep me laughing ... My Dad says I am well trained as I laugh at his jokes ... I can now laugh at my problems, mainly with my Mum and Dad as they know I am a clever turnip.

In 2006 Kate published her own book, *Kate's Story* (Bainbridge, 2006).

Kate's rehabilitation took several years but now, in 2012, she does not have ongoing therapy, without which she feels she is still improving. She goes to a special hotel for people with physical disabilities for two weeks every year and she really enjoys this.

I used to go on respite to Park House, a hotel for disabled people, and it is lovely. They are all so nice and it's a hotel, so nothing medical, but they have nurses and carers 24 hours a day. There, I made lots of progress, like I started brushing my hair and doing my feeds. I know other people think they got me to do my feeds, but I know it was there at Park House. I now go for my holidays there, and I need a holiday after as I do so much chatting and play board games.

I also have been on respite to Sue Ryder (where I met Barbara) and Vitalise but I did not enjoy them so much. There is something about Park House and the fact it is a hotel for disabled people. They have things every night and trips each day.

For a few years Kate went to a day centre for people with brain injuries, at first one day a week and then for two days a week. Initially, she liked going there but there came a time when she no longer wanted to go.

When I left hospital, as I hadn't had an accident, they couldn't find things for me to do. The final answer was joining Contact, where you get university student visitors. A student came each week and talked to me and played board games. I still email ones I had a few years ago; it was a nice way of meeting people.

I went to Headway, but it did not suit my needs, as my memory and mental skills are too good. It did suit me at first as I had to start getting out and doing things. It is a bit of a challenge finding clubs to join.

Now I have joined the WI and the local history group (I did a history degree) and they have interesting talks.

As far as the neuropsychological intervention was concerned, Kate was seen every two weeks for several years to help with her anger and self-esteem. Although problems in these areas reduced, they sometimes reoccurred. In addition, we worked with Kate to help her become more independent outside her home. She learned to go to and from the post box, the library and the cash machine by herself and learned how to cope if her wheelchair became stuck.

I now live in a bungalow with a live-in carer. I talk now, not very clearly, and you have to get used to me to understand me properly. Some days it is better than others, I improve slowly by myself and get no help with my talking.

Another big thing with my recovery is I am very determined and don't give up. I kept persevering for 12 years with talking, then it slowly started coming. I am not really bothered with walking. Although it would be nice to walk, it seems like it would be a lot of hard work! I am trying to stand up, which seems more likely and a bit less hard work.

I now watch funny DVDs, I use my computer lots and read. I have just got a Kindle and I love it. I keep buying books for it. I need to control myself; I say I didn't shop while I was in hospital so I am making up for it. I love shopping and I always have.

I have to mention tiredness as that is a huge after-effect after brain injury, it must not be ignored. When I find people not taking tiredness into account I am very careful if I take notice of what they say. I was OK in hospital as I just sat by my bed doing nothing. Now it is a big thing as I do more. My brain swelling up had a big impact on the amount of work my brain has to do. I can't smell or taste, I have no tears. Also, my cranial nerves got weak so my brain has to work harder to do things like see and hear. When I left hospital I went to Boots [pharmacy] for an eye test, they found my optic nerve was pale. It was such a relief to find that out as I could tell my eyes were not right.

Sadly, my tiredness has not got much better, although my eyes and ears are stronger. Again, it took a few years for my ears and eyes to get OK. My ears still find some things hard, like live pop singing (sounds like they are shouting).

Kate and her parents 2007

Before my illness I liked to be in control. I was happy and I had plans for my life, which have all gone. My illness was a huge shock. I will never get over the shock. My life has totally changed.

In spite of her severe injuries, Kate was beginning to enjoy life again.

I enjoy my computer and emails and Teddy (Kate's cat). Also, for me, having a pet makes me want to stay at home and keep out of hospital so I can see him. Animals don't care what you look like, as long as you do what they want. My parents bought me a kitten when I came out of hospital and that really made me want to stay with him at home. It might just be me, I do love animals, but pets might help recovery and give you a reason to try and stay at home. I think being at home and relaxed are the biggest help to recovery. I like Feldenkrais physiotherapy. I have been having it for five years. It is what Christopher Reeve, Superman, had. The most important thing for me was having a proper assessment and emotional help.

Mrs Bainbridge: *Not to be assessed is like being unemployed, you are not part of the world. It is incredibly important. As a carer, I remember Kate getting incredibly angry with everyone. We didn't know how to cope with it. Family and friends wanted to help and we had to say to stay away, don't visit. We didn't know if it would ever go away. Would I always be torn between my daughter and the rest of the family? The family want to help. They are devastated, too, they say they understand but the hurt is still there. That was worse almost than the illness.*

Kate's father said how angry he became when a doctor once asked him if Kate was always like that – angry all the time. He said, 'Don't you blame Kate'.

The help has made me normal again and brought back my sense of humour. Having people that understood was important. I used to want to die until I got emotional help. We have had to fight for everything. My parents, like me, are very determined – even our cat is. Luckily they support me all the way, not sure I could have made a recovery without them backing me up.

In 2007, Kate spoke of how she saw her life in five years' time. '*I hope mum and dad and Teddy are with me*', she said, but two days later she added to this with an email:

I was thinking about what I want in the future, I really like pets and animals so a dog would be really nice. It would be a friend. I used to have a dog and she was lovely, but very naughty. She used to make me cry. I was her pet! I really miss her and I would like another. I also would like a person to be with me, as you need to fight for everything. I can't see a man ever wanting me as I am so disabled, I will have to have a dog. I never want to live in a nursing home, I like to be in the world.

In 2009, when the first chapter on Kate was published, we said, 'Kate, we hope you achieve these goals'.

Kate 2012

Kate moved in to her own purpose-built bungalow in August 2011 with three carers who take turns to stay with her day and night. She does not have a dog and her beloved cat, Teddy, died but her parents have another very beautiful short-haired British cat, Dolly, whom Kate sees regularly. Kate reads a great deal, she goes to the cinema (she recently saw *War Horse*, which she loved), she goes shopping (she delights in buying earrings), she keeps in touch with a number of people via her computer and leads a full and meaningful life. She said recently that she only screamed when she was unconscious and would not dream of doing that normally. There is also a short film made about Kate, which can be found on YouTube called 'Kate's Story'.

Recovery takes time, so don't give up. I also find I will make progress for a few weeks then I stop. It is as if my brain is having a rest for a few weeks, then I start again doing new things. So my recovery has not been constant – that might just be me, but I doubt it. Also, recovery can take a very long time. I hate seeing on TV people who recover very quickly. I know it is for the time they have in the programme but I fear it may make people think recovery is quick.

My parents were told so many bad things about my case and given very little encouragement, although one nurse in intensive care told my mum, 'Don't give up' and that kept her going.

One final thing, a lady at church said I give her ideas for fund-raising for the church. This made me think that faith has been a huge help for me to keep trying with my recovery. I have lots of time to think and I studied the Reformation at university so I am interested in church history. I find faith helps me keep going as so many therapists have given up on me. They have not said it, but they stopped seeing my recovery because it is far too slow. I hold faith in my mind, I don't shout about it, but feel God and Jesus will never give up on me.

Chapter 6

Jose David's Story

From medical student to medical anthropologist

Barbara A. Wilson and Jose David Jaramillo

Jose David was a successful young man studying medicine when he sustained anoxic brain damage during an operation. After rehabilitation he changed careers and became a medical anthropologist working for the Colombian government. He still uses one of the memory strategies he learned during rehabilitation to help with his work and his everyday life.

Introduction

On 2 November 1995 I was in the third year of medical school in Bogotá, Colombia. I had a score of A for my previous years, and was therefore a successful student. I had been an equestrian competitor since the age of 12, and began riding horses when I was 4 years old. I had also ridden motorcycles since childhood. I was a sociable and friendly person who enjoyed spending time with my friends.

Background of injury

The breaking point of my life

On 2 November 1995, I had an operation on my knee to correct an injury caused by a horse-riding accident. During the recovery period I went into cardiac arrest. This was noticed by the staff who began the recovery protocol immediately, calling for experienced staff to do this. Electroshock therapy was administered to restart the autonomous heart contractions. Nevertheless, records show that cardiac contractions stopped for around two minutes before restarting as a consequence of the resuscitation protocol. I was taken to ICU for 13 days. There I developed an intrahospital pneumonia. On the thirteenth day of hospitalization, it was my twentieth birthday. I was taken to a ward where I spent two more weeks before leaving *hospital. During this time, as well as the care of doctors and nurses, I had, most importantly, the care of my family and friends who were constantly passing by checking the progress. I felt fine, however, and I ignored my real situation. As I left hospital and Christmas came, I had time to study for my final exams that, due to the accident, had been postponed until January 1996.*

Jose David's cardiac arrest led to anoxia in which his brain was deprived of oxygen for an unclear period of time and resulted in injury to his brain.

It was hard to study again. When I read something and tried to recall it, I could retrieve very little. As a consequence of this failure of my memory and attention, I began to change. In January when I got back into university and into the sixth semester, I didn't remember much of what I knew. It was shocking to get in front of a patient to practise a medical exam and not be able to do it correctly because I just didn't remember how it was done. This issue made me ask the school permission to repeat the fifth semester, but to keep the grades I already had from the previous semester. This was in order to have a period to stabilise and remember things once again, and to be in an environment I hoped would help me to remember. However, this wasn't the best decision as I was on a new course with different people who ignored, or had heard the rumours of, my accident but weren't disposed to support me. At the beginning it was hard, but I got used to it. The next semester I asked for a temporary withdrawal from medical school. And more importantly, this stage showed me how important it was to value life. I also accepted my limitations, thus allowing the first stage of recovery to begin.

After suspending his academic studies, Jose David decided to begin a rehabilitation programme, which included speech, occupational and physical therapy. During this period he also saw a psychiatrist for two hours a week. He continued to attend university classes as an assistant in order to test out his ability to learn information, but without formal evaluation.

I have to mention the attitude that my family assumed towards my learning problem. I recall a talk I had with my father who, with his vast experience of industrial and business planning but null on recovery therapies, once said, 'When an engine is broken, it has to be fixed, but in order to have it properly fixed, spare parts have to be changed. What happened to you is probably the same, and as we are unable to change a spare part within your brain, what you need is to acquire the learning mechanisms which can help you cope and surpass your failure, but you need discipline and practice'. Thanks to this, and many more conversations we had, I realised help was needed. At first this was hard to accept, as it entailed many consequences which differed from what I had planned for my life. I had to withdraw from medical school and began a recovery programme designed by a team of health professionals in Bogotá. It was composed of a phonoaudiologist (a speech and language therapist), an occupational therapist and a psychiatrist, all under the guidance of a neuropsychologist named Eugenia Solano. This recovery programme lasted five months. During this time in the morning I did exercise, such as jogging and swimming, on a daily basis. In the afternoon I attended therapy. These therapies were useful as they raised my self-esteem and security within myself.

Phonoaudiological therapy gave the first elements to recover information, such as using quick notes, or making up chains of information so that it could be evoked at the moment needed. On the other hand, the occupational therapist focused on restoring fine movements and decreasing tremors within my hands. The role the psychiatrist played was important as it helped me to understand the stage I was going through; by this time the girlfriend I had at the moment of the cardiac arrest was gone, and this was a moment when I had to look into myself and decide whether to move forward or stay behind, and I decided to move on.

This led to a meeting with the team where we confronted efforts and results and concluded that a more intensive programme was required, and this programme wasn't available within the country. So with my family we decided that I should go to Switzerland, where I had a friend, and learn a new language such as French. We thought that by learning a new language, my brain would have to create new paths of information processing that would also bring back memory and attention, as it was prior to the accident.

Before departing I met another neuropsychologist, Dr Patricia Montañes who, after practising some tests, concluded that although my problem had been surpassed there was still a deficiency in attention, concentration and memory. She mentioned the Oliver Zangwill Centre (OZC), which at that time had recently opened. This grabbed our attention, but the trip to Geneva was already moving on. I moved to Geneva. I was there for two months and went to the OZC for an assessment. When I reached the OZC I was expecting to reach a huge medical centre with many patients and a lot of staff, such as the hospital I used to practise at. To my surprise it wasn't like that, beginning with the town. Ely is a tiny town compared to what I am used to. And the OZC is a place that, although it's small and has few patients or 'clients', has the right staff to attend the needs of them.

In 1997, a Colombian colleague, Dr Patricia Montañes, contacted the OZC to see if we would consider accepting Jose David, a young English-speaking medical student, for our programme. We were concerned that he lived so far away. The OZC is non-residential so clients who do not live locally have to stay in a bed-and-breakfast during the week and return home at the weekend. On balance, however, we thought that the advantages of attending the OZC would outweigh the disadvantages and, after a detailed assessment, Jose David was accepted for a shortened programme of six weeks with follow-up sessions at three-monthly intervals to review progress and set new goals.

Assessment

On my first morning of the assessment, a staff member picked me up at the B&B where I had passed the night. This assessment was meant to evaluate and propose a plan of action for my process. When we reached the centre, I was taken to a community meeting where Jon Evans introduced me to the staff, as well as clients. When Jon introduced me to the staff I was surprised because they happened to be gentle and kind. Jon Evans, Sheila, Claire and Huw were the therapists who conducted the assessment. After this I returned to Geneva for two weeks. During this time the staff at the OZC designed a recovery programme where emphasis would be made on study techniques and short- and long-term memory. They considered that psychological support was required as I was there by myself.

At interview, Jose David said his main concern was his memory and, in particular, learning new information. He reported difficulty remembering things he read and remembering conversations, but his main concern was his difficulty in studying at university level. He said his mood was sometimes low, and at times he found it difficult to accept what had happened to him. However, his scores on the Hospital Anxiety and Depression Scale (HADS) were in the normal range for both depression and anxiety.

The assessments by Dr Patricia Montañes and by the OZC team demonstrated that Jose David had difficulty with both verbal and visual memory and with remembering to do things (prospective memory). There was also evidence of difficulties with attention/concentration and with visuospatial reasoning. In particular, he had problems with sustained and divided attention, together with immediate and delayed recall of verbal and non-verbal material, recognition memory and prospective memory. He was able to apply strategies to learn new material but this was inconsistent and he needed further help with this. Other cognitive skills appeared to be intact: Jose David had good verbal reasoning skills and his working memory (i.e. immediate or very short term memory) was within normal limits.

Neither Dr Montañes nor the OZC team noticed any difficulties with Jose David's speech or comprehension and his social communication skills were appropriate.

Jose David was still in the process of adjusting to his difficulties. Nevertheless he believed that there were some positive consequences of having gone through this experience. For example, he thought he was less self-centred or egocentric and had better insight into what it is like to suffer an illness or disability. Such insight would have been beneficial if he were able to return to medicine. Although he had this better understanding of illness and disability, he also felt there were times when he still denied the extent of his problems. The process of denial is normal and can help the individual maintain a positive outlook. However, as time goes on, it is important for the person with the brain injury to develop a realistic appraisal of the difficulties faced in order to make reasonable plans for the future in terms of work and/or study.

Given that the cardiac arrest occurred 16 months before his assessment, further natural recovery of memory functioning was likely to be limited, so it was recommended that Jose David use compensatory strategies to cope with his problems. He also needed to develop a clear understanding of the nature of his difficulties in order to make plans for his future. Through his work in previous rehabilitation situations and his own efforts, he had clearly demonstrated that he was highly motivated to make as good a recovery as possible. At the time of the assessment, he appeared to be in a transitional phase. On the one hand, he still hoped to be able to restore his memory functioning to its previous high level and to be able to return to his medical studies. On the other hand, he was also developing an awareness and acceptance that this was unlikely to be the case and his life goals needed to be adapted to the new situation. It was, understandably, difficult for Jose David to make definite plans because he was still uncertain as to the extent of further recovery and the extent to which further work on the use of strategies and compensatory aids was able to support his memory.

While still hoping to return to medicine, Jose David was willing to consider economics as an alternative field of study. He spent some time thinking about goals to work on during his six-week programme and wrote the following:

My whole goal is to recover completely from the accident I suffered one and a half years ago but how do I manage to get this? Well that is the question. First of all I'm living a healthy life, which I think is the best for changing in a positive way. I don't drink or smoke and I'm going to start swimming or some other exercise, which I know helps to recover fine motricity. I have always believed that the worst thing I can do is to accept my actual limitations because the day I accept it I will be used to it and won't want to change.

My first aim is to learn a whole new method of concentration and memory, which will be useful for my immediate studies after I finish treatment. Being able to be as fun and spontaneous as I was before ... On this course I'm preparing to get back to college so that when I study I don't have problems with it and I get the results I used to get. I also want to trust myself more than I trust at the moment. I want to learn new experiences with this treatment that will help me in the future. What is more important than carrying out my own rehabilitation, and what is more useful for my future life? I aim to be as normal as I was before and want people to care about me, not because I am like this but because they really love me and like the way I am. I aim to learn how to deal with bad moments, how to take them and how to deal with them. So once again, pack bags, find somewhere to live and move to the UK.

Rehabilitation

Jose David came on to a six-week programme in July 1997 and negotiated his goals with members of staff. The goals and his progress towards them are described below.

Goal 1: Identify his difficulties and his strengths and how these impact on his day-to-day life.
Achieved.

Jose David was asked to make a written record of his difficulties and his strengths and how these related to his everyday life. First, he wrote an account of his difficulties, including the onset of his problems following his knee operation and discussion of his attempt to return to university studies.

For the first three weeks of the six-week programme he was asked to make notes each morning of any examples of difficulties with attention/concentration and memory in his daily life. He was also asked to identify any attempts he had made to cope with the situations and, if he had not coped effectively, to think about whether any other strategy might have been of help. Each of these areas was discussed with a member of the team. Over the course of the programme Jose David became better at identifying problems and potential solutions and was more aware of the impact of his limitations.

Goal 2: Identify the implications of goal number one on a possible return to university. Achieved.

As mentioned above, Jose David wrote about his difficulties and was able to identify some of the ways in which those difficulties had previously prevented him from successfully returning to education. These included study skills, essay writing, following verbal and written instructions and recalling information previously heard. Jose David was able to identify where he had difficulties in these areas and to demonstrate some improvement with the use of compensatory strategies in each of them. During the course of the rehabilitation programme, Jose David decided to apply for a course in London that would allow him to test out the use of his newly learned strategies. He subsequently enrolled on a one-year pre-university course for students from abroad, which combines academic work on a variety of topics, and work on English language.

Goal 3: In a 40-minute period of studying technical material, experience two or fewer attention slips. Not achieved.

The initial assessment work undertaken with Jose David indicated that he experienced significant problems with attention and concentration. Jose David found it difficult to sustain his attention in study situations and was vulnerable to distraction. A programme of attention training was introduced to try to help him sustain his attention. A baseline recording of the number of attention slips during a 40-minute period of studying technical material (neuroanatomy and memory) revealed an average of six attention slips per session. We also used Jose David's self rating of his level of concentration on a 0–3 scale:

- 0 = thinking about something completely different;
- 1 = looking at the material, but not really concentrating on it;
- 2 = attending to the material and trying to concentrate, but finding it difficult; and
- 3 = attending to the material and concentrating well.

On this measure, Jose David's pre-training score averaged 1.6. A further baseline measure was obtained assessing the extent of Jose David's ability to concentrate on a demanding computer task, involving pressing a mouse key as numbers appear on a screen, but withholding or inhibiting responses to the number 3. Jose David's initial performance on this task resulted in

14 out of 50 errors (i.e. failure to withhold response to the number 3). This performance is actually within a normal range, but clearly Jose David perceived his performance as poorer than he would have expected pre-illness. His mean reaction time to the non-targets (i.e. correct presses) was 373.3 ms. The training task involved the use of an audiotaped version of the computer task, which involved Jose David doing the task 'in mind' and mentally responding or not to the stream of numbers on the tape.

Following this training, the full, computerised task was re-administered and Jose David's performance improved considerably, as he made only four errors (out of 50). His mean reaction time had increased a little, to 421.97 ms, and this may represent better calibration of the best time to respond (or not) to the task. However, the mean number of attention slips in a 40-minute period studying technical material stayed the same at six, though Jose David's ratings of his concentration improved. The training therefore appeared to help him to some extent, although not quite to the level hoped. Nevertheless, Jose David felt that his attention had improved somewhat so we then needed to monitor the extent to which he felt things had improved in a real study environment.

Goal 4: Demonstrate effective use of strategies for remembering textual information and demonstrate the use of these strategies on short stories and technical material. Achieved.

Jose David spent a considerable amount of time practising the PQRST (Preview, Question, Read, State and Test) strategy to help him remember written material and demonstrate that he could use the strategy on a wide variety of information, including technical material and stories from newspapers. It was anticipated that the combination of general study techniques (planning and organising study time, preparing for lectures, use of external aids such as a tape recorder), the use of PQRST strategy, and improved attention would increase Jose David's ability to function in an academic environment (though whether this improvement would be sufficient to enable him to cope at university level remained to be seen).

I began my programme learning a new study method, the PQRST (Preview, Question, Read, State and Test), a study strategy that reinforces the key elements taken from what is read, and processed through various techniques aimed to settle the information, and to produce a simple retrieval of information when it's needed. This strategy was complemented through the use of flash cards, keeping an updated diary, setting goals and chain strategy.

For a proper understanding of each of these strategies, a programme was designed. It was then given by various members of staff, each stressing the point of its field of knowledge, and, after having understood the strategy, some tasks were settled in order to measure how much I had learnt. I did my best to make the most of these strategies.

Goal 5: Identify factors that contribute to his low mood. Achieved.

Jose David identified a number of factors that contributed to the low mood he experienced from time to time. In interview, he noted that the major losses occurring in the immediate aftermath of his injury included the break up of a relationship and having to leave college. Issues directly related to his injury included failure to remember information and not being able to function at his premorbid level. He was able to monitor changes in mood by using a mood and thought diary. He identified situational triggers for anxiety and anger (such as buying the correct train ticket, etc) using the diary. He occasionally felt saddened at such changes in his life. This was exacerbated by loneliness on occasion.

Goal 6: Identify ways of coping with his low mood. Achieved.

Jose David was able to identify and demonstrate effective ways of coping with his low mood. In interview, and through supportive group work, he was able to review his current situation, which indicated a willingness to reappraise his life goals. These included accepting that he might not achieve what he set out to achieve prior to his accident. He identified other areas to explore where he might be able to use his strengths, such as going into business. Strengths were high motivation to succeed, and determination, which he had discovered in himself following his injury and had been fostered in defiance of his injury. He identified such activities as exercise, meditation, reading and talking to family and friends, as ameliorating his low mood.

Goal 7: Use an external memory aid effectively at home and at the centre. Partially achieved.

While Jose David was initially rather reluctant to use any form of external memory aid, he agreed to use a Filofax when it became evident to him that he found it difficult to remember to do things and remember future events. By the end of the six-week rehabilitation programme, Jose David demonstrated good use of the Filofax in the centre. However, it was felt that he required further work in this area in order to use the method effectively for managing many aspects of his daily life.

Being at the OZC wasn't just to get some strategies. It was getting the idea that I was recovering, by various activities that are held within the centre. One that must be mentioned is the community meeting. This is the space where staff and users get together in order to discuss issues that are expected to arise when people share common spaces and have the determination to recover. Also, the psychological assessment provided is important. When being at the OZC and getting to comprehend what a disability entails, a person has to receive psychological assessment. A third component was provided by the Understanding Brain Injury group, a space where it's said what a BI means, and provides elements to cope with your specific accident. In my case, this was important as I had the previous anatomic knowledge of the brain, and was able to make proper anatomical and physiological relations. A fourth component entailed fine motricity therapy and movements, which normally is a consequence of BI. All these areas brought together made the OZC experience an unforgettable one.

Jose David engaged well throughout his six-week rehabilitation programme and demonstrated progress in a number of areas, as outlined above. He enrolled on an economics course in London, which gave him the opportunity to test out the work he had completed at the OZC. We recommended to Jose David that he attend the OZC half a day each week in order that we could continue to help him to apply the strategies he learned and identify new ones where appropriate.

Another thing that should be mentioned is that, during the time at the OZC, I began to exercise physically in my spare time. The Ely sports complex turned out to be the place where I trained. I attended the pool at seven and swam until quarter past eight. At nine I went into the OZC where I stayed until half past three. This was followed by a session in the gym until six and then back home to get some sleep and be waking up at five every morning. It turned out to be a way of living, which, as a consequence, modified my interest. During this period the 1997 economic Asian crises arose. This created an interest of knowing what was happening. I decided to study in detail the crises, and therefore applied to study economics at the School of Oriental and African Studies (SOAS), part of London University, where the experts in Asia were able to provide thoughtful explanations for the origin of the crises.

Further goals were set with Jose David for the next three months.

Goal 8: Demonstrate transference of study skills from the rehabilitation environment to his college course. Achieved.

Jose David was able to transfer his PQRST strategy to his college work. While he could not apply the strategy in every study situation (because of the pressures), he was able to use it as a mental guiding model to help direct his work. Jose David demonstrated effective essay planning skills, including time management. He learned to organise his lecture notes effectively and manage his time well in relation to study time and planning for lectures. He was waiting to take mock exams in March 1998.

During the year at SOAS I kept contact with the OZC on an email communication basis. I attended the centre twice for a one-day visit where I held meetings with my therapists and was able to inform them of my progress due to the methods learnt at the centre.

A report was received from one of Jose David's college tutors that said the college was pleased with his progress and noted that he had a serious attitude towards study and a genuine intellectual curiosity. Furthermore, Jose David had considerable confidence, and was perhaps, at times, over confident in his abilities. Jose David recognised the amount of work he had to do on both his English and other courses in order to do well, and he had responded appropriately to this.

Jose David felt that he was more successful on this course than on his previous attempts at returning to University. He believed this was due to three main areas: being on a more structured course; his own confidence; and the treatment he has received (including his homeopathy, the rehabilitation programme at the OZC and his self treatment).

Goal 9: Identify any needs he has relating to his mood and report these. Achieved.

Jose David continued to keep a record of mood rating in his diary; there was no change since the last report, i.e. his mood remained stable. He maintained a positive outlook while remaining aware that he might not achieve his ultimate ambitions.

Goal 10: Identify a plan for future actions with regard to his studying/rehabilitation. Achieved.

Jose David decided to return to Colombia and consider either a return to his university to study medicine or a change of course.

Outcome

Fifteen years have passed since I left the OZC and, after having studied economics, anthropology, holding a master's degree in Medical Anthropology and looking forward to doing a PhD soon, I can say it was a time well spent, probably the best investment done in my life.

I still use the PQRST without the T strategy for tasks that need to be accomplished within my professional career. In my personal life, planning is important and I use it daily now without even noticing, it has become part of me. I got married in 2009 to a lovely woman, whom I love. We had a baby girl in October 2010 and those are now the most important things in my life. I'm currently working as lecturer in Medical Anthropology at a university in Bogotá, and have done various researches on health issues such as 'teenage pregnancy myths' – completed for the health council of Cundinamarca's department, and 'corruption within the public health of Colombia' – for the controller's office of Colombia. For my dissertation in my undergraduate degree in anthropology, I conducted research on traditional healing remedies for malaria on the Pacific coast, and the dissertation for the master's degree was on 'Narratives of HIV patients in Bogotá'.

Barbara and Jose David met up in Bogotá in February 2012. He looked very well, was happily married, and a father.

For those who read this account and are in a similar condition yourself, or a family member, the suggestion I can provide is to keep faith and maintain a discipline to recover. Constancy and decisiveness will provide for rehabilitation to happen.

Chapter 7

Tracey's story

Quality of life with locked-in syndrome

Barbara A. Wilson and Tracey Okines

Tracey was a young mother who worked part-time in a children's nursery when she had an accident one day in the gym. The symptoms became worse over the next few days until she went into a coma and it was discovered that she had torn an artery deep in her brain. She survived but was diagnosed with locked-in syndrome, a condition whereby people are fully conscious and intellectually intact but in which they can only move their eyes. Despite being almost completely paralysed, Tracey leads a happy life.

Introduction

Before my accident I was a confident, energetic young woman. I worked part-time in a children's nursery. I loved my job. I had the energy to keep up with the children and I never suffered from headaches so the noise never bothered me. I have a daughter. She was six years old when I had my accident. I lived alone with her.

I did part-time modelling. I was always told as a child that I was ugly and that I could never be a model so I had low self-esteem. I was an ugly duckling that grew into a swan. I was more interested in playing football and climbing trees than having boyfriends. That was until I was 14 years old and hormones went raging. From the age of 14 I have been single for about two months. I was attractive and I knew it. I was one of those cows who ate whatever I wanted; I never dieted and never went a size over eight.

I had a little puppy, I loved taking him for long walks, and on my days off work I would go for a jog with him. I also loved doing yoga and dancing. I would give most physical activities a go. I would be the first on a dance floor, I wouldn't shy away from a party. My friends called me the life and soul of a party. My parents always moaned at me for burning the candle at both ends.

I loved shopping and buying new clothes. I loved fashion. I enjoyed painting, I found it to be a relaxing hobby. I did like cooking but I wouldn't say I was particularly good at it.

I saw my parents about once a week. I moved out of home when I was 17 and I was very independent. I was a working single mum who didn't drive so I couldn't visit my parents a lot more than I did. Besides, I had an older sister who lived near to them. She didn't work, and visited my parents a lot. I loved my parents but I talked a lot and my views differed from theirs so I felt like an annoyance.

I got with Joe in October 2007. He was a male version of me. My friends said we were very well suited. We met at art college when I was just 18 years old. But for some reason we had never got together.

Background of injury

On the evening of my accident I was going to take my daughter swimming. I had packed our bags ready. Joe phoned and there was a gymnastic taster session in my gym and his uncle would be going so we decided to go there instead. We waited for Joe to finish work. We went to the gym and we were asked to cartwheel across the room. As I did this I lost my balance and fell on my head. My head didn't really hurt but my ankle swelled up like a balloon and was agony. I told the gymnastics instructor what had happened. She ushered me away and told me it was my own fault for being silly. I got home that night and bathed my foot in cold water. I had presumed I had just sprained my ankle. The next day I attended work, my ankle still hurt but I was hobbling about. That evening I attended my friend's Ann Summers party at her house. A lot of the girls from my work would be there. We finished looking through the catalogue, then I went outside for a cigarette. But when I went back inside I had an agonising pain pounding through my head and I felt dizzy. I sat down before I fell down. The dizziness went but the pain continued. My friend gave me some painkillers. I later went home to Joe.

I launched myself into his arms, tears rolled down my cheeks. He put me to bed and I fell straight to sleep. Apparently that night I had a fit. Joe never told me, I was none the wiser. I don't remember much of that weekend. Along came Monday. I don't remember this but apparently I went to the doctor where he sent me home with headache tablets. That evening I went salsa dancing with Joe and his uncle.

My friend had taken her daughter and mine to McDonald's. My ankle was hurting but I hobbled through the activity. After the dancing I picked my daughter up and tucked her into bed. I went into the front room with tea where Joe and his uncle were sitting. I had a pain go through my head and neck. Joe gave me a neck and shoulder massage. I don't remember what happened next. I just remember lying face down looking over the side of the bed into an empty sick bowl. I think I remember Joe shaking me by the shoulder shouting, 'Tracey, snap out of it, you are having one of your funny turns.' I don't remember what happened next. Apparently I was having a fit. Joe called an ambulance but I heard they were called way too late to save my mobility.

Whilst in hospital I was stabilised and given a drugs test, using a strand of my hair. It showed traces of drugs in my system. When questioned, my friends lied and said I'd never taken drugs in my life. They thought they were helping me by lying but they were making my situation worse. The medical staff just presumed I had taken a drug overdose. My daughter had told my father I had fallen in the gym. My father told the medical staff but they wouldn't listen. Over three days later I was given a CT scan. They realised there was something wrong in my brain and I was sent to Hurstwood Park. There they put a camera in a vein in my leg. It went to my neck where it stopped. That was when it was realised I had damage in my neck. The injury was done in the gym, as my father had been telling medical staff.

I was on morphine so I was a bit confused with reality and dreams. I remember the room being dark and I could hear sirens outside. People ignored me and talked like I wasn't there. I felt a bit confused as to why it had happened to me. My dad explained what had happened. Mum and Dad knew from the start that I could understand them. Some of my carers believed this too, but some did not. I felt completely guilty that those who cared for me would have to see me in such a state.

Then, as I came round from the morphine, reality hit and I realised everything was true. There is no point in me being angry as it won't change anything. I've just got to make the most of a bad situation.

Tracey's MRI scan showed that she had suffered a basilar artery thrombosis. A neurologist confirmed that the fall in the gym had probably caused a tear in the inner wall of the artery, which in turn caused clotting in the brain. Tracey went back to the original hospital where her parents were told she would probably not survive for more than a few months.

The MRI scan found a large lesion in the pons (a structure in the brain stem). Some 90% of the pons was affected with slight sparing of the extreme posterior section. The mid brain and thalami were not affected. There was no evidence of lesions in the cerebral hemispheres, particularly in temporal or parietal areas. Mild to moderate generalised atrophy of the cerebral hemispheres was seen, together with moderate atrophy of the cerebellum. No hydrocephalus or other intracranial abnormalities were found.

I had gone into a coma in Hastings; there was little hope that I would come out of the coma. I stayed in intensive care in Hurstwood Park for two weeks. Then I was transferred back to Hastings. I was in a coma for about four weeks. A lot of people thought I was brain dead but a nurse noticed my eyes were watching her as she went past. The staff would talk to each other thinking I couldn't understand them. I could. I learned a lot of gossip. I received a lot of cards from well-wishers. Many contained empty promises of forthcoming visits. Only a few handfuls of people actually visited.

After a month in the coma, Tracey began to regain consciousness. About four weeks later a nurse noticed that Tracey's eyes were following her as she moved around the room. Tracey's parents were told that their daughter was aware but her cognitive state was not known. A diagnosis of locked-in syndrome (LIS) was made. LIS is a rare consequence of brain damage. The condition is typically caused by a lesion in the pontine area (in the brain stem), usually a stroke in the basilar artery or a pontine haemorrhage. According to Schnakers *et al.* (2008), at least 60% of all cases fit this picture. Patients with LIS are fully conscious but unable to move or speak due to paralysis of nearly all voluntary muscles except the eyes. Communication is with movement of the eyes.

I woke up one morning and my whole life had changed. I get treated like I am stupid. It's patronising. People cannot bother to use the (communication) board as it takes too long. It's frustrating. At the beginning no one knew I could understand and they would talk in front of me. I found out loads of things I shouldn't know. At the beginning I thought I was in a computer game and my aim was to hide from the nurses.

I never did see Joe again. I'm not sure what happened to him. I just woke up and he was gone. When I awoke from my coma my whole life was completely different. My daughter was living with my sister, my dog was living with my friend, a stranger had my job, everything in my flat was taken to the tip. I never saw a lot of my friends and boyfriend again. I was more angry than upset. I had enough to worry about without thinking about other people.

I battled against a lot of illness in hospital. I battled against chest infections, urinary infections, thrush of the mouth, excessive sweating, hair loss, weight loss, vomiting, foot drop, depression and many more. After three months my sister decided that she couldn't cope with my daughter so, without talking to me, she put my daughter into care.

As Tracey became more alert she was able to answer questions by raising her eyes for 'Yes' and lowering them for 'No', allowing her parents to communicate with her. Her father accessed the internet and found information from the French locked-in syndrome association (www.alis-asso.fr). A letter board was described using colours and letters. With some modifications, a similar board was made for Tracey, and this is how people now communicate with her. The chart is organised with different colours on each row. Each row has certain letters and numbers. Thus, the first row is red and this has the letters A, B, C, D and 'end of word'; the second row is yellow and has the letters E, F, G, H and 'new word'; the third row is blue with the next set of letters and so forth. The last two rows are white, depicting the digits 0–9.

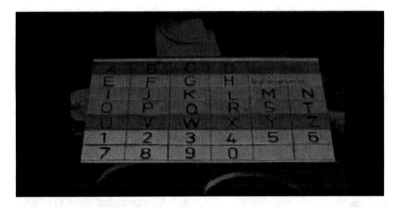

Figure 7.1 Tracey's communication board.

First, Tracey is asked to select the colour red/yellow/ blue/green, etc. When Tracey raises her eyes to the right colour we then say the letters (or digits) along that row until Tracey raises her eyes. Words are spelled out in this way. Tracey is very good at this. She does not need to actually see the board nor do those who communicate regularly with her as they can remember the colours and letters, but it is needed by others less familiar with the system.

After five months the hospital said there wasn't any more medically they could do for me. I was sent to a neuro-rehabilitation unit in Salisbury. I was lonely there but grateful not to bump into anyone I knew. It was here I saw my reflection for the first time since my accident. I was very upset and didn't like it. I was very ill here and spent a lot of time in hospital. I suffered from fatigue and spent a lot of time in bed. I thought if I spent my time asleep then the time would go quicker. A nurse told me that having locked-in syndrome meant that I was going to die.

I stayed there for about five months, then I moved to a place in Tonbridge. Some people would like it there. I hated it. The staff were foreign and didn't have good English. I've nothing against foreign people but when you have communication problems being around people who don't speak the same language as you is hard.

The biggest battle was boredom. I used to get sat staring at a wall or a tree out of a window for hours. We weren't allowed radios or television. I wasn't liked because when I was told I wasn't allowed something I asked why. I wasn't allowed make-up, my own decorations or anything electrical that could help with my communication. And I had to have alternative medication. I nearly lost my personality here. I was so miserable.

After 21 months I moved to a place in Hastings. I got a lot more visitors, I went out a lot more and got a lot of my confidence back. A friend told me that people weren't blanking me because of the way I looked but because they did not know how to cope with my disability. I realised it was everyone else's problem not mine. All my carers were English so they didn't just understand me, they also understood if I was making a joke. Because my confidence increased I saw changes in my physical being and I am doing a lot more.

Assessment

Tracey has a tracheostomy tube in place. She is fed by a peg tube and she has hardly any movement apart from a little facial movement of her tongue and lips. This allows Tracey to make a small smile and she has limited head control. She is, however, alert and engaged.

At a first meeting in January 2010, her father, John, and her speech and language therapist showed us how to communicate with Tracey using the letter board. The referral to a neuropsychologist was to determine whether or not Tracey had any problems with her memory, concentration, thinking and so forth. We knew about locked-in syndrome (LIS) and had assessed people who communicated with a letter board, but had not assessed someone with LIS before. Tracey was always cooperative and appeared to work to the best of her ability. She was seen two or three times a month until June 2010. Assessment was slow because of the communication method Tracey is forced to use (eyes raised for 'yes' and lowered for 'no') and certain tests, such as tests of speed, motor functioning and recall of long passages could not be given. Nevertheless, many tests could be administered to her. It soon became apparent that Tracey had good concentration and an excellent working memory. She rarely forgot what word or sentence she was spelling and could keep in mind instructions given to her.

As well as tests of reasoning, memory perception and other cognitive tests, Tracey was assessed on a test of anxiety and depression, a scale to measure her perception of pain, and a test measuring her quality of life.

Tracey did well on most tests. On two tests of executive functioning (problem solving and reasoning) she scored in the superior range of ability. This was also true of a test of verbal memory. She was good on tests of naming and language as well as basic visual perception and visual spatial processing. There were two areas where she appeared to have some difficulty: the first was in some aspects of visual memory and the second was with some more complex visual perception, visual organisation and visual reasoning tasks. This was thought to be due to the fact that she has some diplopia (double vision), and blurring of vision, making it difficult for her to scan complex arrays. She says her vision is 'like looking through the window of a moving vehicle with bad suspension'.

There was no suggestion that she was depressed or particularly anxious and Tracey, herself, agreed with this when the scores were fed back to her. On a pain rating scale, Tracey said she could feel pain normally anywhere in her body; she rated her headaches as 85 on a 0–100 scale and said she had this pain about four times a week. The pain was described as 'heavy and severe'. She believed her headaches were caused by her posture and a visiting pain expert said she thought this explanation was probably correct. Tracey's head is supported in a headrest, but due to her decreased head control and her strong cough reflex, when she coughs her head will fall forward causing increasing strain on the neck muscles. Since the pain assessment, Tracey has had rest breaks during the day and this has reduced the severity and frequency of her headaches.

On the quality of life measure, Tracey felt her general health was much better now than a year ago and she was experiencing far fewer respiratory infections. She did not rate herself as having any emotional problems and believes she has a reasonable quality of life. Emotionally, Tracey would appear to be a well-balanced young woman with no serious cognitive difficulties and no obvious depression, anxiety or other mood issues, despite the severe limitations placed on her because of her almost total paralysis. With Tracey's help, we wrote a paper about LIS that was published in 2011 (Wilson, Hinchcliffe, Okines, Florschutz & Fish, 2011).

Other people with LIS

One of the world experts in LIS is Steven Laureys from Belgium. In 2005, he wrote with his colleagues an excellent chapter called 'The locked-in syndrome: What is it like to be conscious but paralyzed and voiceless?' (Laureys *et al.*, 2005). They say that the earliest report of a patient with LIS in the medical literature comes from Darolles in 1875. Even before that, however, Alexandre Dumas had described the condition in *The Count of Monte Cristo* (1844).

The best known case of LIS, however, is probably that of Jean-Dominique Bauby, who 'wrote' *The Diving Bell and the Butterfly* in 1997. Bauby had a brain stem stroke in 1995 when he was 43 years old. He could only move his left eye. He wrote the book with the help of an amanuensis who used a frequency-ordered alphabet, which she recited aloud. Bauby blinked his left eyelid when she reached the correct letter.

Unfortunately Bauby died shortly before the book was published. In 2007 a highly regarded film was made of his story.

Two other books by survivors of LIS are *Look up for Yes* by an American woman, Julia Tavalaro (with co-author R. Tayson), also written in 1997 and *Only the Eyes Say Yes* by a French couple, Philippe and Stephanie Vigand (2000).

Julia Tavalaro had a haemorrhage in 1966 and was comatose for seven months, during which time she was placed in long-term care. She gradually regained consciousness but it was not until six years later that her condition was correctly diagnosed. Her mother and sister believed Julia was aware for years before a speech and language therapist, Arlene Kraat, worked out a way of communicating with her. In the book, Tavalaro writes movingly of her pain and distress in the years before Arlene Kraat and an occupational therapist began to change her life. She used her eyes to tell of her terrible years 'in captivity'. Eventually, she was able to use a communication device and wrote poetry. Julia died in 2003 at the age of 68 from aspiration pneumonia.

Philippe Vigand had a stroke at the age of 32 and was in a coma for two months. His wife realised he was communicating by blinking his eyes in response to her questions but she had difficulty convincing the staff. One day the speech therapist was assessing Vigand's gag reflex. Vigand bit her finger, the therapist yelled and Vigand started to grin. Thereupon, the therapist asked, 'How much is 2 plus 2?' Vigand blinked four times. A letter board was then used initially until Vigand went home and was able to use an infrared camera, which was attached to another camera allowing more sophisticated communication. The pair discuss Philippe's LIS from their different points of view. The book was published in 2000.

Garrard *et al.* (2002) describe a woman who developed LIS after a visit to the hairdresser where she had held her head backwards over a sink. She became unwell but it was five days before the full syndrome appeared.

A rugby player from New Zealand, Nick Chisholm, had an accident on the rugby field. It took three days for his condition to deteriorate and for the diagnosis of LIS to be made (Chisholm & Gillett, 2005). Several other papers describe patients where it took several days for the full-blown condition to appear (e.g. Allain, Joseph, Isambert, Le Gall & Emile, 1998; New & Thomas, 2005).

As with the patients described above, the striking finding from Tracey's history and other reports is the very slow onset of the stroke leading to the LIS. It was several days since Tracey's original accident in the gym until the full-blown paralysis and, again, as we have noted, this is true of several other patients reported in the literature. The patient described by Garrard *et al.* (2002) who had been to the hairdresser's suffered neck pain, nausea, dizziness, clumsiness of the right arm and dysarthria and then, five days later, a full-blown stroke developed. These symptoms were very much like those described by Tracey. Other cases in the Garrard *et al.* (2002) paper also showed slow onset.

Perhaps the case most similar to Tracey was a 37-year-old woman who developed neck pain after slipping while standing on her head during yoga. Three days later she became paralysed and anarthric (unable to speak). Most other strokes would appear to be of a much more sudden onset.

Conclusion

What lessons can be learned from Tracey's experience? We have to say first of all that Tracey's spirit and sense of self are admirable. Despite some shocking misunderstandings and lack of attention from those in charge of her in the early stages, she remains determined and does not fall into self pity. She reacted well to our testing and, although she seemed to relate well to some of the people who worked with her at the centre in Tonbridge, she was bored and some people found it difficult or too time-consuming to communicate with her so she feels less than positive about her time there. One positive thing that happened is that Tracey's chest infections decreased. She said when interviewed at the Tonbridge centre that she thought one of the positive aspects of her life since her accident was that she did not get so angry at small difficulties any more as, in the grand scale of things, these were not important. Sometimes she was frustrated because people could not be bothered to communicate with her, and sometimes she felt fearful because she could not see what was going on around her but basically, she just had to get on with life.

In 2005, Laureys and his colleagues said that most able bodied and healthy people thought that life with LIS would not be worth living. This is in contrast to what most people with LIS actually feel. Despite some recent highly publicised cases, the Belgian group (Laureys *et al.*, 2005) and others such as Anderson, Dillon and Burns (1993), Doble, Haig, Anderson and Katz (2003) and Smith and Delargy (2005) found that people with LIS typically report a meaningful quality of life. Smith and Delargy state: 'The finding that locked-in syndrome survivors who remain severely disabled rarely want to die counters a popular misconception that such patients would have been better off dead' (p. 409). Tracey certainly has a zest for life.

Chapter 8

James's story
Returning from the 'dark side'

Fiona Ashworth and James Mallyon

James was a burn-the-candle-at-both-ends kind of guy who lived life to the full. His slaughter factory job involved long hours and intense physical labour. He balanced a tough job with a passion for partying, loving heavy metal and living an alternative way of life. You could say he was an 'adrenaline junkie'; one of his favourite activities was getting out on his motorbike. This life dramatically changed the night he crashed his motorbike on his way home from a night out; his candle-burning days were over.

Introduction

Now aged 43, James has spent all of his life in a village near Cambridge. He did well at school, particularly in subjects he liked including art, woodwork and metal work. After leaving school, James was employed in a meat production factory where he worked his way up the ranks and became a slaughter man. During this period, he lived in an annex of his parents' home. He enjoyed his job and working with his peers, describing himself as someone who 'worked hard and played hard'. He lived on the edge: he kept boa constrictors and tarantulas as pets, attended festivals and concerts, went clubbing and rode his motorcycle fast.

Before the accident, I was definitely happy, contented in the life I had. Pretty much did what I wanted to do. I didn't have to give it a second thought. I very much lived in the moment. I still had to work, pay taxes etc., other than that if I wanted to disappear I could do. I was like an old hippy (without the beard!). The work life – a slaughtering job, it was tough but I really liked the people I worked with and it was very social – I loved going to festivals, concerts, going abroad. I did lots of stuff – motor racing, darts, clubbing – I was out most nights. I felt comfortable wherever I was. I was pretty confident, not bothered about making a fool of myself In fact I was quite happy to make a fool of myself! I was just who I was – living on my own but not secluded.

Background of injury

The bike accident. I should never have been on that road, particularly on the bike I was on. I'm pretty hazy about what happened. I was on a bad road, I knew it was bad. I decided to use the road that night; I went round a corner, saw the deer in the road and chose to miss the deer in that split second. I thought it was a flat edge on the road, but it wasn't, it was a ditch. That's when everything changed. My next memory was crawling out of ditch. I felt lots of pain and was confused; I think the adrenaline took over. I thought I better ring mum to get the neighbour's van. I phoned mum, there was a lot of fussing – told her to get Norm to come get me. I still thought at that point that I was fine, that there was nothing seriously wrong.

After the accident, quite a few people were coming down the road and they stopped, included a mate who stopped as well as some other friends and strangers too. It seemed like there was a lot of people. Then the pain really started to kick in. I didn't really know what happened after that – I was told the police turned up and then an ambulance arrived. I remember a painful trip in the ambulance on a stiff board.

No one knew how long James was unconscious, but it was probably under an hour. He was conscious when the ambulance arrived and he was admitted to Addenbrooke's Hospital where doctors found that James had suffered extensive injuries, including a fractured clavicle and ribs as well as a brain injury. No MRI or CT scan was done at the time of admission. There was no evidence of retrograde amnesia, indicating that James probably experienced a mild traumatic brain injury (TBI). He was discharged home with a prescription of 30 sessions of outpatient physiotherapy.

I was in hospital for five to seven days, in intensive care for two days. I don't know exactly how long I was in hospital for. Then I went home to my parents – biggest mistake I made. Not because of my parents, but because I was sent home so soon. I thought that if I went home I would be okay, at the time I wasn't in pain because of all the morphine I was on. It was stopped when I left hospital. I had terrible pain and headaches then, I had to take painkillers all the time – 16 during the day and 16 at night. This went on for months – actually I had headaches for at least a year.

When I was at home, I had no contact with anyone. My sleep was not good; it was erratic, some fitful sleep during the night or during the day or both. Then I saw the neurologist and he said I had depression, it all came to forefront. I had only gone to see him for the headaches. If I hadn't gone to see him I don't know where I would be now.

During the first two months at home, James was mostly immobile, spending time between his bed and a chair, after which he began to use crutches. Two months later he was able to walk short distances without the crutches, but he struggled to cope with the physical pain of his injuries. Five months after his accident, James was seen in the neurology clinic for a brief neuropsychological assessment, which highlighted slowed information processing, poor memory and symptoms of depression. Around this time, in late 2008, James attempted to return to work on light duties. However, the factory he worked in closed down and he was made redundant. He took part in a 'Pathways to Work' scheme but was deemed medically unfit to work.

Assessment

In March 2009, James was referred to the Oliver Zangwill Centre (OZC) by his neurosurgeon and seen for an Admissions Assessment in September 2009.

Cognitive assessment

Prominent impairments were found on tasks of attention and speed of information processing. James's performance on memory tasks varied as a function of the amount of processing undertaken, so that he had trouble remembering information presented quickly and in large quantities, but was able to remember better when he had the chance to study and learn. Tasks involving greater cognitive demands could lead to mild executive difficulties including goal neglect, disorganisation and difficulties problem solving.

Psychological assessment

James found it very difficult to adjust to the consequences of the TBI, and as a result he had both depression and anxiety. Furthermore, he showed cognitive and social communication difficulties that exacerbated his psychological distress. James himself said that he had trouble remembering both to do things and how to do things and could not organise himself or keep track of his goals in the moment. He felt low and depressed and had lost his confidence in social situations with others, which led him to feel very anxious. He was worried that he did not know what he could do for work anymore, but it was important to him to be able to find a vocation and return to work.

In summary, the assessment highlighted cognitive deficits that interacted with and impacted upon James's mood and behaviour and affected his ability to effectively pursue functional goals such as work and social activities. Formulation of James's difficulties was conducted using a variety of assessment processes integrated into a biopsychosocial framework (see Wilson, Gracey, Evans & Bateman, 2009).

Rehabilitation

James attended rehabilitation at the OZC (see Chapter 1 for programme description) where he identified some key areas that he wished to work on. He wanted help with his memory and with returning to work and, although he felt depressed, he still lacked an overall awareness of the extent of the cognitive, communication and psychological difficulties resulting from his TBI.

Coming to OZC for rehab. There was a lot of . . . I don't know . . . as if you are standing back and watching but not taking part. I was turning up but not really taking it too seriously, really I was blagging it and denying so I was resisting a lot. It was partly to do with the stuff around the brain injury and partly to do with other people which changed my mind – we (peer group) were all talking about the same problems, the same issues, especially when someone says 'I cried at the TV' – I did that all the time too! Then I just accepted it and grabbed hold of OZC and the staff in both hands. It really helped to have time to be able to talk to the other clients without the staff there.

During the early part of the programme it was evident to us that James was struggling to engage with the rehabilitation process as he was resistant to ideas and seemed distrustful of the staff. However, it was clear that he had committed to the programme as he attended every day. Therefore, the first and most important goal for us was to build a good rapport with James; evidence within the field of clinical psychology practice indicates that a good therapeutic alliance is the key ingredient to change (Lambert & Barley, 2001). As highlighted in the first chapter of this book, the therapeutic milieu is key to the process of holistic neuropsychological rehabilitation and we felt that this would also be a catalyst for helping James become more engaged in the process (James's peer group consisted of three other clients: two young men and a middle-aged woman all having experienced a TBI). In combination with this, the team utilised a motivational interviewing approach (see Miller & Rollnick, 2012) to support James in moving through the five stages of change (DiClemente & Prochaska, 1982) in order to help him gain greater benefits from the rehabilitation programme.

At this point in the rehab, when I decided that there was something I could do, I thought, 'okay, I have to fix it'. It was probably about two months or so into the programme. But then I went downhill – they call it a 'U-bend' at OZC, there are millions of ways to describe it. It definitely set me backwards. I was still in denial, you see I had always been very independent, never asked for help – I just don't do that. I thought to myself, 'I'm going to fix it, not someone else who had read books and s**t.' But then I started to realise that they knew what they were doing, I had to try to let go, almost like handing over, I had to learn to ask and accept help. I'm not used to asking so it was tough.

As James became more engaged in the process, he started setting key goals related to the areas he wanted to change. As is common in interdisciplinary team (IDT) work, the team worked jointly on his goals, although different professionals took the lead in those areas related to their expertise.

Goal 1: James will develop a shared understanding of the cognitive, communication, mood and functional consequences of his injury

In the first step of this programme, James and his team developed a shared understanding of the cognitive, communication, emotional and functional consequences of his TBI through Understanding Brain Injury (UBI) groups, including Cognitive, Mood and Communication Groups and individual sessions. For example, common difficulties with psychological adjustment after brain injury were discussed in the group sessions with his peers and those difficulties personal to James were discussed and formulated in one-to-one psychotherapy sessions. This process was repeated for social confidence, cognitive and communication problems and functional difficulties.

As part of this process, James developed a UBI portfolio. He reviewed his medical records and physiotherapy notes and pieced together the events early after his TBI. He also challenged some unhelpful beliefs he held about certain events, which he may have been informed about incorrectly or recalled incorrectly. In this way he was able to establish a clearer narrative of the events surrounding his TBI and develop a better understanding of what had happened to him in order to adjust to and move on from the injury. By the end of the intensive phase, James had a clear formulation of the difficulties he was experiencing as a result of the TBI. He demonstrated this through his written portfolio of the consequences of his TBI and description of how these consequences interacted and affected each other.

James has a great talent for drawing and he began to use this skill as part of the rehabilitation process, including drawing a picture of his experience of his brain injury through the process of rehabilitation. This drawing depicts his journey to date and was begun during the rehabilitation process and completed after he finished the programme (see Figure 8.1). James describes moving from initially a sense of being out of control after the injury and in a 'dark place' to feeling able to take back control of his life through rehabilitation, depicted by the spiral of experiences being held in the palm of his hand. The use of art in brain injury rehabilitation is felt to have many therapeutic benefits, as described in a BBC documentary (Hammond, 2010).

Armed with a better understanding of his injury, James was now ready to move on to learning strategies to manage and compensate for the consequences of his TBI. He was determined to develop strategies for (a) managing his depression; (b) improving his social confidence; and (c) managing his memory failures and executive dysfunction.

Goal 2: James will learn strategies to manage his depression

Working together with James, the clinical psychologist took a lead in working on the depression, whilst the speech and language therapist (SALT) took the lead on improving social confidence.

The psychological formulation highlighted that James had been struggling with depression and generalised anxiety, including lacking social confidence. High levels of self-criticism were a key factor maintaining James's psychological difficulties since his TBI. He described this self-criticism as an inner voice, 'a screaming voice, shouting at myself or getting angry with others.'

James and his psychologist agreed to use an adapted Compassion Focused Therapy approach (CFT), which is specifically aimed at working with mental health problems such as depression and/or social confidence issues in order to reduce the emotional and social impact of self-criticism

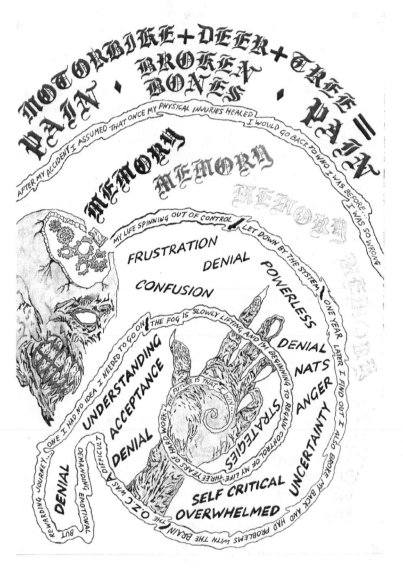

Figure 8.1 James's depiction of his journey through brain injury rehabilitation.

(Gilbert, 2005; Henderson, 2011). This approach has recently been used for those with TBI (Ashworth, Gracey & Gilbert, 2011).

As James found it particularly hard to describe his feelings and emotional experience in words, he began to share his emotional experiences through drawings, which depicted particular points in his journey since the TBI, which he described as the 'dark side' of life. These drawings were used as part of the psychotherapeutic process, and an example of this can be seen in Figure 8.2 depicting James's early experiences of depression after his TBI. He described this drawing as an inner self-portrait stating, 'This is how I felt other people perceived me after the brain injury, I felt somehow like I wasn't a nice person anymore.'

Furthermore, given that James struggled with verbal descriptions, behavioural experiments were also used as a key part of not only the psychological work but also all other rehabilitation efforts (Bennett-Levy et al., 2004).

Key to the psychotherapeutic work was the introduction of compassionate mind training (CMT; Gilbert & Irons, 2005) to aid James in managing his self-critical response to the changes he experienced as a result of his brain injury. As he was experiencing severe depression, his psychologist referred him to a neuropsychiatrist in the belief that a combined approach of anti-depressants and psychotherapy would be most beneficial. The psychiatrist prescribed anti-depressants and, although James was initially ambivalent, he chose to try them as a 'longer term behavioural experiment'.

Overall, James made slow but significant progress in overcoming the depression. At the end of the programme, James's self-report measures highlighted a reduction of symptoms of depression as measured by the Hospital Anxiety and Depression Scale (HADS; Zigmond & Snaith, 1983). During a recent review, he also told us that he was feeling much better in himself, and although he still faced challenges, he was more able to manage them.

Mood sessions and the 'dark side'

Even though the emotions were not really there, emotions were the hardest – very overwhelming at times as well. I would never have talked about that, it was a new experience as I was trying to adjust to a new way of coping as well as a brain injury. In the beginning, I thought, 'Am I changing who I am, or is who I am being changed without my control?' And because I didn't like the changing I could resist. It was almost like I could see a video of myself, shouting at me to change but not being able to do it.

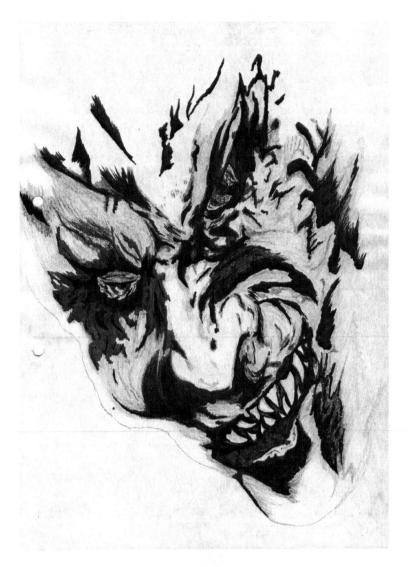

Figure 8.2 James's depiction of his 'dark side' after brain injury.

Things changed gradually, it wasn't overnight. There is no defining moment. It was a slow process. I think it was the inner voice. Instead of screaming at some-body, or myself, it began to analyse. Rather than screaming uncontrollably, it (the inner voice) became strong but not screaming. The voice started to then mellow out a bit. After that, I liked that I wasn't crying so much, I really didn't like the crying from before. This is when I knew there was a significant change. There was a part I noticed and I thought, 'This is me getting better'. Something was happening, and I felt a lot better in myself. Then I started to think about what else made me happy.

Goal 3: James will learn skills to increase his social confidence and decrease social anxiety

James's lack of social confidence left him anxious in social situations. In addition to psychotherapy aimed at reducing self-criticism, he worked with his SALT to improve his confidence and reduce his anxiety in social situations. The SALT collaboratively set up a number of behavioural experiments with James to increase his communication confidence, including chairing and presenting news items in the centre's daily community meeting as well as starting conversations with unfamiliar staff at the centre. These experiments were set up in a graded hierarchy. James learned strategies to increase his confidence in communication, including planning ahead, role-play in advance and thinking about possible scenario outcomes. Each experiment was reviewed afterwards and James reflected on his levels of confidence and anxiety after each one. Over time, his social confidence in communication increased and his anxiety reduced. He continued to work on the graded hierarchy after the programme. James still finds some social situations challenging but feels he has the tools to manage them.

Goal 4: James will learn strategies to manage cognitive difficulties in day-to-day life, both at home and at work

Unsurprisingly, James's cognitive difficulties impacted significantly on his everyday life. Work in this area was conducted jointly between James's occupational therapist and his psychologist. His psychologist focused on developing awareness of the cognitive challenges and strengths he had, followed by developing compensatory strategies to manage these challenges. The OT supported James in putting these compensatory strategies into action in his everyday life in order to help him to manage more effectively. She helped him develop a memory and planning system that enabled him to plan and complete activities consistently. She also developed a vocational action plan (see next section) which meant that during the integration phase, James did a work placement in a tattoo parlour. The placement provided opportunities for testing out strategies. Initially James was ambivalent about using strategies because, prior to his TBI, he had not used any type of strategy (e.g. diary, calendar or notebook).

Cognitive testing for rehabilitation planning had identified difficulties with speed of information processing, attention affecting new learning, and executive functioning including planning and goal management. As James became more engaged in rehabilitation, he identified managing at work as his main goal for cognitive sessions. He learned a number of compensatory strategies to help him be more effective at work and at home. Again, the behavioural experiment approach was used to test out predictions relating to difficult situations at work and use of strategies. Through this process James set the following specific goals:

(a) Being able to learn and remember the correct steps involved in new tasks at work

James learned to use an errorless learning approach (Wilson, Baddeley, Evans & Shiel, 1994) in cognitive sessions. Initially, he used post-it notes placed discreetly next to the equipment he needed to use at work, outlining the steps in order that each task was achieved. Over a number of weeks James reported that this worked well for him and he generalised it to other equipment and tasks where necessary.

(b) Being able to keep on track without losing sight of the main goal using Goal Management Training

James was introduced to goal management training (GMT; Robertson, 1996), adapted for his needs. This involves employing a '*STOP, define the main goal, identify steps, learn the steps, and check outcome*' self-talk strategy. James commented that, over time, this system enabled him to keep better sight of the main goal and go off track less, although he did continue to struggle with this. We gave him a key fob with a bright red 'STOP–Think' as a visual cue to remind him to 'Stop–Think – What's my main goal?'

(c) Being able to be more aware of time in order to use it more effectively

James noticed in the work placement that he was not noticing time passing and would think that less time had passed than actually had (e.g.

when one hour of actual time had passed, James reported it to be about ten minutes). He felt this impacted on his work, particularly towards the end of the day when he had a number of the same tasks to complete but would often not leave enough time, or would start very late and not be able to finish. James found that having an alert on his phone at a certain time in the afternoon (e.g. 3 pm) reminded him to start his end of the day tasks on time. Combined with a clear laminated tick list of the tasks to be completed, the alert supported him in getting the tasks done. Although he found this useful, James still struggled to perceive time correctly.

(d) James will develop a memory and planning system to manage his correspondence at home

His occupational therapist worked closely with James on expanding an external memory and planning system in his home so that he could be more organised. By the end of the programme, James was using a notebook for his 'to do' list and a correspondence file to manage his correspondence at home (as after the TBI he was not opening letters consistently).

Goal 5: James will explore his work skills and opportunities of pursuing a career as a tattooist by completing a work placement in a tattoo parlour

James had always been interested in the art of tattooing and had many tattoos himself. This passionate interest led him and his team to consider the possibility of his working as a tattooist. With support from his OT, James began a placement in a tattoo parlour – despite his attempts to get the OZC staff to have tattoos as part of his vocational plan, none of us took him up on the offer!

James's boss, tattooist George, communicated openly and honestly about the difficulties he observed. James set about testing out strategies to help him overcome these challenges at work, as described above. The voluntary work took place on Thursdays, Fridays and Saturdays and amounted to just under 16 hours per week. A phone review was arranged half-way through the placement, and a face-to-face review was held at the end. The feedback was positive. George felt that James did the tasks asked of him to a good standard, although he acknowledged there were some areas in which he needed more support and strategies. For example, it took James longer to learn new information, such as using the steriliser machine. This was an example where using an errorless learning approach incorporating the step-by-step how to post-it note worked well in helping James overcome the cognitive consequences of the TBI.

George felt that James's performance during the placement, together with his artistic skills, indicated that he had potential to pursue becoming a professional tattoo artist and offered him a 12-month apprenticeship. It was agreed that he would continue to do the tasks required of his placement together with learning the principles and techniques of tattooing on a voluntary basis. He was also put in touch with the local Disability Employment Advisor who would support him after the programme.

My work

She (OT) really helped with my job; I think it was a little exciting in the beginning but mostly there were dark feelings. There was a lot of darkness surrounding it for me. When I first started there was a lot of acting involved, if you don't show it they won't know. I can be myself now at last. I am not putting on a brave front. There was a lot of acting and pretending initially. I am working in a tattoo parlour – I remember getting the wrong transfers – lots of the time! But now I really do enjoy it, I do have some of the same problems but I have things to help and also a good sense of humour!

Outcome

Since finishing the programme, James has been working as a paid tattoo artist with George. He thoroughly enjoys the job and feels he has good 'banter' with his boss. Recently James returned to the OZC as a mentor, to offer advice to newcomers to the programme. He talked to a group of seven clients and two staff members and another group of approximately seven clients, two staff members and nine family members. James reflected that he felt very comfortable doing this and could remember the first time he had spoken in a group early in the programme and how difficult it had been. He said,

I will never forget that first day talking in the community meeting, I was thinking why the f**k am I doing this? I was feeling so uncomfortable, but I did it, and each time I did it and thought about it after, the better I felt. Now I feel really comfortable talking in front of a group. In fact, I really enjoyed coming today and would like to come back and do it again.

My general reflections

Life is hard – before the brain injury I didn't realise how hard it was. I always used to have a sense that life is easy, but now I realise how hard life is ... But the difference is, although I still struggle with a lot, the time spent struggling is worth it, it's worth the struggle and heartache. I can feel physically sick all day sometimes, I didn't have that before. If I didn't have rehab at OZC I don't think I would have been anywhere close to where I am now. It's had a massive effect on my life now and my family. It's hard to explain it when you are there all day though – it is tough, but it was very important for me to talk to other clients. It was one of the hardest things I went through, but I feel like inside it was one of the best things that ever happened to me; as sick as it sounds it's like climbing Mount Everest – when you reach the top, you achieve it. I felt so alive like nothing else, it was a similar sort of feeling getting to the end of rehab but actually rehab never ends, it just slows down.

My message to other survivors

I think it's important to open yourself up to the rehab – you'll regret it if you don't! Learn to accept that rehab can help. Even if you are not certain, try it out for the duration. Talk to other survivors. I also noticed other people (survivors) changing from the first to the last visit – we were different at the end, I can't exactly explain how. I remember one of the other clients in my group saying at the end of rehab, 'We are different people now'. I felt happier, more confident.

My message to health professionals working with survivors

Anyone can experience this (the brain injury), you can experience it yourself. You can only really know what it's like if you experience it yourself. The only people that know it are those people who have been through it. I think it's important for the staff to know that the journey never really ends. This is the journey. I would tell health professionals who work with survivors like me to really listen and have patience. Patience is key. It really helps when they have patience, and also when they try to understand and show empathy, that's really important.

Chapter 9

Claire's story

A face is not a person

Barbara A. Wilson and Claire

Claire, a 45-year-old mother with four children and employed as a nurse, developed herpes simplex encephalitis, which left her with a number of cognitive problems, the most severe of which was prosopagnosia, an inability to recognise faces. This meant she could not recognise her husband, her children or her own face. Despite this, Claire continues to lead an independent life.

Background of illness

Claire was admitted to hospital with herpes simplex encephalitis. An MRI scan reported a high signal intensity in the right mesial temporal lobe, extending into the adjacent basal ganglia, insula and inferior frontal lobe. Limited high signal change was also evident in the left temporal lobe. Claire was unconscious for about a week. We first got to know her when she was referred to the Cognition and Brain Sciences Unit for a neuropsychological assessment. Neuropsychologist Bonnie-Kate Dewar worked with Claire for several months and continued to see her when she went to the Oliver Zangwill Centre (OZC). Claire was found to have prosopagnosia, an inability to recognise faces. This is a rare and handicapping condition which, in severe cases, means people cannot recognise their own faces or those of the people nearest and dearest to them. This was true of Claire, who did not recognise her own family. In addition to face recognition problems, Claire was found to have impairments of memory, word recognition and retrieval, verbal abstraction, speed of cognition and visuospatial skills. She had a further assessment to investigate her facial recognition difficulties in more detail.

There are very few treatment studies of prosopagnosia but the consensus seems to be that it is difficult to treat. Personal experience suggests that people with prosopagnosia typically have to compensate for the deficit in some way, for example, by recognising a person by voice or by a distinctive piece of clothing or jewellery. As we were unsure whether it might be possible in some cases to restore the ability to recognise faces, we decided we should attempt restoration in the first instance. Photographs and semantic information were collected of family and friends whom Claire had difficulty recognising. Following multiple baseline assessment, eight faces were selected for training. Instruction in face identification was practised with the aid of a mnemonic and by using the errorless learning paradigm of expanded rehearsal. Two faces were presented at weekly sessions, in addition to home practice. Recall of all faces was tested at the beginning of each session. Although Claire learned to name the faces correctly following training, and was also able to recognise the same person when a different photograph of that person was shown, this improvement did not generalise to an improvement of face recognition in general.

Claire's difficulties were made more severe because she found it hard to recognise people from their voices and therefore preferred people to wear name badges or to tell her who they were.

Assessment

Claire was referred to the OZC to see if she could benefit from our rehabilitation programme. Accompanied by her husband, she attended for a one-day preliminary assessment. She reported that her main problems were low confidence, anxiety, depression, poor facial recognition and organisational difficulties. Her anxiety took the form of shaking, tearfulness, headaches and pins and needles.

Rehabilitation

It was felt that Claire would benefit from the programme on offer. The next step was a two-week detailed assessment before coming for the full programme. Claire's rehabilitation programme was considered a success and, although she continues to have considerable difficulties, she lives independently, travels on public transport, does some voluntary work and engages fully in life. Indeed, Claire has some extraordinary abilities that seem to have remained intact. These include her remarkable insights into her own problems and subsequent analysis of the various rehabilitation treatments and techniques she has experienced and practised with a number of therapists; her understanding of her situation in regard to her own family and the new life she leads as a result of the difficulties caused by illness; and her outstanding ability to analyse and write coherently about her difficulties. In view of these exceptional talents, it has been agreed editorially that Claire should have her own voice in this chapter and provide the reader with her own account of her struggle to come to terms with the lifetime consequences of encephalitis.

Claire's thoughts

I consider myself to be a very lucky person to be a survivor of encephalitis. I know that many other people have been nowhere near as lucky as me. Firstly, I was in the UK when it happened, and in the most advantageous place in the postcode lottery as well. My husband is a doctor and realised promptly that I needed urgent hospital care – apparently I called him 'Stephanie', which confirmed the need to take me to hospital! So I was treated efficiently and early and have had excellent medical care throughout. I am a survivor of the illness but sadly not of its lifetime consequences. It has altered the person that I am, and I'm not able to call myself 'me' any more. My parents have a daughter who doesn't know them. My husband has a wife who has completely changed personality, who has lost her feelings of belonging to him, and our children have a mum who doesn't know them, can't support them through life and who struggles to remember how to be a mum.

But I've survived physically, mentally in many ways – and I'm learning how to manage with some damaged bits. I have been extremely lucky to have had a huge amount of support and understanding from my family and friends, and very high quality holistic neuropsychological rehabilitation from the best suppliers of this service that anyone could ever wish for.

What happened to me

I was a busy working mum, happily married, with four healthy, happy children, then aged 8, 10, 13 and 15, two boys and two girls, not forgetting the rabbit, the snakes and the cats!

I have no memory of what happened but I am told I'd had a couple of days of being unwell with a temperature, cold/flu like symptoms and a headache, and became increasingly confused. Apparently, I was behaving quite oddly and my family was becoming worried about me. I was taken to our local hospital and quickly treated with medication, and then I was transferred to intensive care at a larger hospital some way away. I had slipped into a coma by this time. I was diagnosed with herpes simplex viral encephalitis and treated with IV Acyclovir. The virus had somehow managed to cross the barrier from blood to brain and caused severe inflammation of the brain tissue. I am told I had seizures at this time.

I remained in a coma for five and a half weeks, and am told that many kind people visited me in this time. Thankfully, somebody made me a visitor's book, and kept all my 'get well soon' cards, which are very precious to me now. I wasn't able to thank them, or know they had been to visit me, which has been very upsetting since. Ed brought our children to visit me regularly and I have lovely notes kept from them. It was at one of those visits that I'm told I made my first meaningful word after all that time unable to respond. One of our sons spoke to me from a place I couldn't see him and I said his name: 'Leo'. They must all have been so delighted and relieved, just to know that 'I' was still there – wife, mum, Claire.

The eleven weeks between then and my discharge home are also unrecorded in my memory and I feel absent from such an important time in my life, and still have very little understanding about what happened whilst I was in hospital. Ed has told me that one day he was feeding me, and offered me a piece of cauliflower (which I love) on a fork. I leant forward and kissed it! I was awake in hospital feeling very lost, confused and disorientated in my surroundings. I had awoken into a world I knew nothing about. The first I knew about anything was being told I'd had a virus six weeks ago. I know that it was some time before I had any concept of the consequences of the illness myself. I didn't initially realise that I was unable to recognise or remember anybody's identity. I had bad dreams regarding people's identity during that time.

So what did that mean to me? Here I was, being told that I was somebody who I knew nothing about, that this man 'Ed' was my husband, and that these four children were ours. I knew nothing about any of them and couldn't recognise anybody. I had no understanding of my life, where I lived, worked, or who I shared it with. Words can't describe just how lost and confused I felt. My family were strangers to me, whatever it must have been like for them I can't imagine. It was very hard for me to accept that these strangers were my family. I think I was able to believe that the children were mine, from a strong maternal instinct but it was very difficult to feel the same confidence to re-bond with Ed. I told myself to believe that as I had married him, that this man must be the right man for me, even if I didn't know anything about either of us anymore.

I started to see the neuropsychologist who explained how and why my autobiographical memory was so severely impaired, why I had such profound amnesia about my life and why I was struggling so hugely to encode new memories of what was happening then. She helped me to understand the consequences of my illness and made me feel that it was normal, accepted, expected, and all right for me to feel so awful. She helped me to accept my changed circumstances to some extent and together we worked through valuable ways for me to adjust to the changes.

In hospital I had been able to relax and was supported in understanding and managing life little by little, but when I was discharged and at home it was completely different. It felt as though I had crash-landed into somebody else's life, one where I was meant to fit but I just felt so lost and separated from the whole thing. I came home to a house I couldn't find my way around and, although I wanted to do the usual household tasks which I had always done, I didn't have a clue where to start. My family were strangers, I didn't know where anything was, or how to get around the house, and for a long period of time I was very scared. My family made notes for me, and lists and made sure they told me how to help them properly and were very kind and understanding when I needed help, or did things wrong. I found pink heart-shaped post-it notes all around the house to help me: 'Bedroom', 'Bathroom', 'Tea bags', 'I love you mummy', amongst others.

I didn't know myself or anyone else. I couldn't recognise animals/birds either and even now, eight years later my family still remember and remind me happily that I named everything as a giraffe! I had no concept of gender, initially, and had to re-learn ways to appreciate this, and also skin colouring confused me too. I get startled by mirrors and don't even recognise myself in them. Going into the department stores in the city centre was, and still is, hard as I struggle to realise that the dressed up models aren't real people. I jump out of my skin and feel very wary in that environment – even little hedgehog planters in the garden centre shock me.

The first New Year after I was home, we all went as usual to the New Year's Eve party in the village hall. I was very anxious about going, knowing that I wouldn't recognise anyone, that I'd struggle to keep with Ed and/or the family and that lots of people would say happy 'Hellos' to me and greet me as the friend I used to be. I still very much want to be their friend but that's very hard when I don't know anything about either of us anymore. One of my kind friends brought name badges for everyone to wear. The names alone didn't help me very much, but they announced my difficulties to everyone and I did get lots of hugs!

Prosopagnosia tends to be initially described to people as 'having no facial recognition'. Sadly, it's much deeper than that; not only do I not recognise somebody's face but I struggle to have any memory of their identity. I don't know anything about them, anything about their lives, how we know each other or what parts of our lives we have shared. They're a stranger to me. When they happily tell me their name – 'I'm Sally!', 'I'm Linda!', 'I'm Christopher!' – they think that's enough for me and they feel happy that I'm reminded who they are. But a name isn't everything. How many Lindas do I know? Have I worked with a Sally? Is Christopher my son? A name doesn't give identity and not having the helpful prompt of recognising someone's face leaves me panicking about who this person is, and how to react to them appropriately.

Following discharge home I continued to have outpatient appointments at the hospital. Every meeting with the psychologist was very valuable to me, and it felt very secure being in the company of somebody who really understood and cared. And she wrote and posted a letter with everything we'd covered, and our plans of action, which arrived in the post the next day! 'See your social situation as something you can manage rather than something that controls and overwhelms you.' It was fantastic to have it written, and I felt very secure about the advice and support being safe. I could re-read it whenever I liked, and still do now. She made me feel safe, that my reactions to what was happening were normal, and her great words, which gave me much strength, were 'together we can'.

My home life and social life were both very stressful and, despite all the support I was having, I continued to feel very upset and confused about life generally. Everyone was helping me, which was great but it made me feel useless and rejected – rather left out of a life I was trying to re-find. It was hard enough for me, but it must have been terribly complicated for my poor family. Ed needed to take over more home/life responsibilities and parent our children almost alone as they grew through their teenage years. He has stayed very understanding and caring for all of us and has held our family together.

Rehabilitation at the OZC

I was referred for continuing neurorehabilitation at the OZC. My needs were assessed, I began the programme with three other survivors of brain injury and we completed our rehabilitation together.

Barbara Wilson spoke to our group and said these words, which enabled me to think and feel quite differently about my progress – 'Rehabilitation is not synonymous with recovery'. Wow! That turned a huge corner for me. I understood that I was rehabilitating, not recovering, two completely different concepts that I hadn't realised I was mistaking. I then was able to tell myself that we have one life, and that we must live it, and here I was being given all the support and strategies to manage the complications in mine, giving me the ability to help myself to live it happily. No one can do it for me, I have to do it for myself, no one can mend my brain and I knew I was being given a real chance during my rehabilitation to appreciate my difficulties and learn ways of supporting myself, and to rehabilitate!

We had group sessions to give us information about brain injury generally and these allowed us to appreciate and understand our own problems and also each other's. My notes from that time say 'sense-making sessions, and in 12 weeks we should be experts in our own brains and the consequential changes in our behaviour'. UBI (Understanding Brain Injury) group sessions helped us to understand and to focus on ways we do manage and helped us to keep sight of positive ways we manage to help ourselves. We also had Cognitive Group Sessions to appreciate all manner of invisible difficulties in everyday life, understanding the concept that the computer, or controlling part of the brain, is the cognitive side, and it is this part which helps us to operate effectively.

We had Psychological Support Group sessions together, forming goals to become supportive of each other. One day we chose to discuss voice intonations together and changed pronunciations of things to give altered meanings. I learned a lot from this session, and we all had a good laugh! We also had sessions for a Mood Group, which I can't remember much about, and my notes only say something about hot cross buns! Seems like we were in a very good mood – which we were all the time during our sessions as it felt so supportive and relaxing to be there together.

We had Leisure Group outings, which we organised together, all supporting each other in having separate responsibilities towards them and ensuring that we recognised each other's difficulties. Meeting these helped the events go well for each of us. We enjoyed a lovely walk around the town centre one day and I have some lovely photos to prompt my already lost memories of a really great day. We did Strategy Application group sessions together to identify our different skills, any difficulties with these and to find strategies for management together. Each meeting we appointed a chairperson to run the meeting and a secretary to take notes, print and supply them to each of us to keep. At the end of each meeting we had feedback time to evaluate if our aims had been achieved, what had gone well and what we would do differently next time.

My family and friends have had a very difficult time living with all the complications of my illness, and complete personality change, and they too have gained enormously from my rehabilitation. They were also given information about my difficulties and how to support and to help me themselves. They were included in the rehabilitation programme with family and partner sessions as much as they felt was needed.

During the second three months of the programme, the Integration Phase, I was given support to do some voluntary work. I was very anxious initially but the placements were given information about me and they were able to understand and give me appropriate ways to help, to enable me to manage and to increase my own self worth.

The group sessions were very advantageous to all four of us and we all gained very much from the whole concept of how difficult even simple things became for each of us. We were able to learn together and value each other's improvements as well as our own. We also had Communication Group together where we were able to learn about how we communicate with other people and skills for how to improve our own difficulties with this. We all became better able to understand and respond to social situations in a more meaningful, social way to establish and maintain friendships.

Life since the Oliver Zangwill Centre and what I am like now

Barbara has asked me to talk about my life now, and before I start with all the practical chaos I just want to say that I am feeling much more secure about my life now as I am using many strategies to guard and record my memories, which is giving me a new sense of security about them. I had started to do photo-scrapbooking when our children were small and have many treasured albums, some home videos of those times and hundreds of boxes of extra photos still to do. During my rehabilitation I felt supported to go forwards and have been happily recording my new memories but am very emotionally upset about attempting to cope with my lost ones. But I'm getting there! I'm now eight years on and busy sorting all my boxes, albums and files of memories, feeling very secure now that they're mine, belonging to a real me and that I can share and feel part of them whenever I'm ready to. They're safe. Memories are very special and we must guard them, treasure them and feel happy sharing them.

My memory problems haven't changed. I still have the same large memory loss and difficulties making and storing new memories: semantic memory for facts; autobiographical episodic memory for things that have happened; and prospective memory for future events, planning etc. I have problems with my topographic memory – where places and items are; my olfactory and gustatory memory for taste and smell has been damaged and I have difficulties learning new informa-tion. My greatest challenge is the prosopagnosia, the face-blindness and identity uncertainty of all people, including myself, which has left me living in a world full of strangers, with no sense of belonging.

One day recently I'd been to my aqua-aerobics class where I enjoy exercising in the pool with a group of other ladies. We were all back in the changing room and I suddenly realised that one of them was looking at me. I caught her eye and tried to decide if she wanted to speak to me, or if I was expected to remember something, or know her? I glanced away to gain a second breath, and then looked back towards her to see if she was still making any social contact with me. I saw that she'd also looked away and was then making eye contact with me again. I was unsure if she knew me or not or whether she was going to say anything, and she looked uncertain about whether she was going to or not. I began to feel rather uncertain about this person and worried that I possibly seemed aloof and unfriendly towards her as she was clearly trying to connect with me in some way, but just not being sure made me hope that she'd make the first social inter-action so that I may respond if I needed to. We looked rather uncertainly at each other several times before somebody walked between us and I suddenly realised that it was a mirror! And I had been looking at me! No wonder she was looking so confused.

Prosopagnosia – it's a big word meaning a world of strangers. Communication between people begins with many decisions when we come into contact with each other. We see body language, facial expressions and general demeanour/manner, listen to spoken word and during this time we are ascertaining the identity of this individual. For me, it's a face, and it could be anybody. Their facial expressions are what I try and use to ascertain whether they are individuals supposedly known to me. Humans have a myriad of facial expressions, which change extremely quickly and body language and mannerisms can say a lot about what they are thinking. We can't read people's minds but that is almost what I'm trying to do each time I look at a face. I am trying to read their unconscious messages they're virtually unintentionally giving me. What I want, and need, to know very quickly is whether they know me, and then, how well, and in what circumstances do we share parts of our lives together? I need a lot of reliable information in those few immediate seconds, from seeing the face, and very specifically from making eye contact, to ensure that I respond appropriately to them.

For instance, I want to be able to greet my husband with wide eyes, a big smile and a hug but I don't wish to behave in this way to a man in the village post office who happily greets me. A face isn't a person, it's a series of expressions which I need to see to attempt to read the messages they're giving me, and I struggle to have confidence to react appropriately in all social interactions. I have spent much time guarding these difficulties by not making eye contact with people, unless they speak to me first and say who they are (and preferably how I know them). This has prevented me from hugging the wrong people and embarrassing both of us, but it has also made me seem shy, uncaring and aloof to others. Eye contact usually then involves some expectation of words, speech may begin but there follows the next round of complications and uncertainty. These vary from one extreme to another – we may completely ignore each other and not be even remotely interested in any way, or there may be the big hug, huge smiles, kisses and complete sharing of feelings together, and about each other. I need a lot of reliable information in those few immediate seconds, from seeing the face, and very specifically from making eye contact to ensure that I respond politely/appropriately to them.

My confidence for social interactions being manageable depends very much on the time and the place – whether I'm expecting to meet up with anyone in particular or not, also depending on how many other people are also around me at the time. It's very common for people to greet me happily and tell me who they are, which lots of people do now, and the ones who know me well enough to know that their name won't be enough for me do give me some extra information to help – 'I'm Jo, your Glastonbury friend!', 'I'm Pat, the egg-man!' – and of course it's normal for me to meet people in places other than where I expect them to be, which is even more confusing for me. When I do say to people that I'm not sure who they are I regularly get, 'Oh yes! I never remember names either!'.

I realised early on that I needed written information about people's identity to allow me easy access to know who they are, how I know them and what parts of our lives we have shared. I made myself an A to Z identity book, a friendship file and many notebooks to help me with directions and home-like commitments as well. All these have helped me hugely but I am trying to live a life which doesn't feel like it belongs to me anymore; it has dramatically changed, not just for me but for everyone around me. I knew so many people and shared friendship, the access to which I have now lost. I feel lonely and a failure to everyone around me.

I don't feel able to be the wife, mum, friend, daughter, sister, nurse who I think I was before. Everyone around me has their own conceptions of this person I have to call 'me', this person I seem to be, but nobody knows me and nor do I. I live alone in somebody else's life, but I am living in continual contact with people who do know lots of information about the person I was, and their knowledge and happiness sharing their memories sadly compounds my feelings of loss. I have felt very lonely in their company and have needed to resist hearing their happy stories about times in our lives which feel so empty to me. I feel very sad to have lost the real warmth of sharing memories with friends, and even though I feel I'm getting hugs as the person I was rather than who I am now, I do feel that they are still my friends and I'm trying hard to rebuild my understanding of who we all are.

As I began to gain back my confidence to travel by public transport again, I started to attend open meetings run by the Encephalitis Society [www.encephalitis. info], interested to see if they had any new ideas about how I may manage things better. Their meetings were very informative and everyone was made to feel very welcome and cared about. We had plenty of free time between sessions to relax and talk to other people, and one day I began chatting with another lady who was also there all by herself. She asked me what my main problem was, and when I said prosopagnosia – she said so was hers! We made an instant friendship and have shared our difficulties together and given each other much understanding and support which has been really wonderful. How fantastic to suddenly meet someone else with the same problems. She even gave me the right word for the flavour of sweet things which I no longer liked – 'metallic'. I'd always said 'sour' but knew it didn't quite describe it right. So there we were, both unable to recognise each other and both of us unable to be the known person who we both needed when out in social situations.

Initially we met up in very specific places using pieces of paper cut out into the shape of a jigsaw piece each. I had the red piece and my friend had the blue piece, matching the jigsaw pieces on the logo of the Encephalitis Society showing two pieces of life's jigsaw fitting back together. At our meeting place we would both be checking for somebody holding their paper piece, or having it next to them at a coffee shop somewhere – and it worked! We have since bought a bag of loose beads and made ourselves matching necklaces which we now wear when we are meeting together, and needing to stay together. A bit easier than our jigsaw pieces and we look a lot less bizarre to the onlookers.

The concept of life's jigsaw being broken was helpful to me and best when I'd finished my rehabilitation at the OZC and our son, Struan, said to me that we had found the four corners now and we were rebuilding the sides so we could throw all the pieces back into the middle.

Four years after the illness I was asked if I would help with some research work testing a new piece of equipment, which it was hoped would help people with memory problems. Over a period of months I wore the SenseCam and recorded events also written into a diary. The SenseCam is a small camera worn around the neck which takes photos with a fish-eye lens every 20 seconds or at any change in light or movement. The SenseCam loads the photos into a computer where they can be seen rather like an old home video, and although each photo is an individual shot, they do sequence very well. I reviewed these photos and my written notes at given intervals and the researchers did their testing about my memory capabilities.

Right from the beginning I was able to know that the event reviewed from the SenseCam later gave much better triggers to my memories than my written notes. The photos weren't the standard 'tall at the back, short at the front, and SMILE!' photos, but very meaningful snaps of every moment, completely unstaged and they gave me a real sense of having been there, being part of it, and belonging. And the feeling of security of my memories has been the best bit. They're safe, in the computer, and I can turn them on and re-live them whenever I like. The researchers' results showed that the SenseCam cues stimulated my episodic memory well, concluding that consolidating memories with the SenseCam led to more retrieval of new information, in particular sensory-perceptive details and cognitions, giving me a feeling of 'being there' and 'reliving'. They felt that, although I was unable to consolidate new memories, the SenseCam imaging bridges this gap for me, allowing me to feel part of my own life. Looking over at my SenseCam images feels very special and I'm told that it stimulates what little remains of my episodic memory. It felt great that the researchers were pleased with the positive results and an fMRI scan proved that this was right as my memory areas lit up with far greater activity when I was asked to think about events previously reviewed on the SenseCam.

Technology is evolving fast and I am one of the first brain injury patients to benefit from this fantastic new device. I'm also happy now that it is now marketed as a Vicon Revue for others to use and to give real security to their new memories. One of the researchers described my feelings about it as a 'Proustian moment'

– that 'a rope had been let down from heaven to draw me up from the abyss of unbeing'. And after the research I was allowed to keep it!

Now, a further four years later, I have thousands of SenseCam memories, all mine, to re-live whenever I want to, which gives me a huge new sense of security of belonging to my own life. I look back over them to remind me about times, events and people involved. I have a notebook with me at all times which I use to write notes about where I am, what I'm doing and who I'm with so that I have a written record to know which of the thousands of pictures are going to trigger my memories. I have some great footage of doing a Charity Challenge – fundraising for the Encephalitis Society, Trek Transylvania which my new friend through the Society and I did together, with our necklaces on! And she had a new Vicon Revue then and since we have had great times sharing our memories together – who was first to the top! Who went over the bridge when we were meant to climb on stones through the river! Memories forever.

Finally

I think of myself as a very lucky person who has survived as best I could have thanks to my wonderful family, and all the wonderful people who have understood and supported me throughout. Crossing life's bridges hasn't always been easy but I've had lots of help to paddle through the river and step on stones to help me to get to where I am now. And I'm using my SenseCam to record me tripping and falling, but also succeeding, to throw all the pieces of my life's jigsaw back into the middle with great relief. I am re-finding 'myself'. My body is fine, my brain is rehabilitated and my 'being' is becoming clearer each day. Thank you especially to Barbara Wilson as I see her as the integral cog in my rehabilitation and feel very privileged to have been in the right place at the right time for the postcode lottery of life.

Chapter 10

Jason's story

Putting a spanner in the works

Fiona Ashworth and Jason Corfield

Jason is a gentle, kind and humorous man who is committed to doing the best for his seven-year-old son Joshua. He takes great pleasure in the simplicity of life, particularly enjoying nature. In fact, he grows bonsais and has a real passion and love for nurturing and caring for them. He is a creative man who also enjoys carpentry and shows great skill in this area. Jason's life was changed forever by a series of strokes at the young age of 34.

Introduction

Jason is a 40-year-old man who was born and raised in Peterborough. His parents and younger brother live together not far from his flat. He is very close to his father who had his own haulage business. Jason was a well-behaved child whose favourite subjects at school were the sciences, maths and catering. He left school at 16 after studying mechanical and electrical engineering as well as carpentry and joinery. He worked in the carpentry industry until he was 21 when he was made redundant and then moved into the food industry. He excelled in this area and was promoted, but he chose to return to carpentry as he found the food industry too stressful. He worked in a boat building company as a carpenter. Jason married at 27 but divorced seven years later, soon after his strokes occurred. His son Joshua is now seven years old. Jason is a proud and honest man who was always busy prior to his strokes.

Background of illness

The journey started some five and a half years ago, when I had three strokes over a 48-hour period. Prior to that, I was a busy family man, with a young baby. I worked really hard to provide for my family and to give my son as many experiences as possible from such an early age. I was a carpenter and joiner, working for a very well-known luxury boat builder (Fairline Boats). But then all of a sudden it's like falling off a lorry, or like hitting a brick wall with the effects it's given me for the rest of my life. But at that time I didn't realise how much impact the effects would have.

The strokes happened two days after Jason received physiotherapy on his neck for what he believed was a trapped nerve. MRI and CT scans indicated damage primarily to Jason's cerebellum, indicating a right posterior artery stroke, although it is likely that other areas may have been damaged as a result of loss of oxygen to the brain. On admittance to hospital, Jason had a PEG fitted due to dysphagia. He spent two weeks on an assessment ward before moving to the stroke ward, where he spent a further three weeks.

After the strokes I gained a condition named Wallenberg Syndrome, which left me with poor balance, nerve damage plus poor cognitive function, fatigue and poor mood. After the strokes, the cognitive functions affected included processing speed problems, plus attention issues and memory problems. My mood was also affected with depression, low self-esteem and anxiety.

Wallenberg Syndrome, also known as Lateral Medullary Syndrome, is relatively rare. This caused Jason a multitude of symptoms including weakness of his right arm and leg, reduced pain sensation in the top of the right side of his head and in his left foot, altered temperature sensation, and pain in the right side of his face, which is worsened by cold, nausea, dyspepsia and reflux.

Jason attempted to return to work, but was unable to do so due to the consequences of his stroke. An occupational psychologist at Job Centre Plus assessed him and found some cognitive difficulties. Jason struggled to cope with the impact of his strokes, he soon became depressed, and eventually his marriage broke down.

Jason was prescribed medications to reduce the risk of stroke, to manage neuropathic pain, and for depression, reflux and nicotine cessation. Following an appointment with a Specialist Registrar in Rehabilitation Medicine, Jason was referred to the Oliver Zangwill Centre (OZC).

Initially, I was beating myself up a lot in the early days, even in hospital. I was also avoiding things, avoiding the truth of how serious it was. I was in quite a lot of denial about the effects. I was having quite a lot of problems: I couldn't sleep; I was having sleeping problems, although the hospital did say to rest your brain you need to sleep. I was also afraid of not being able to be the dad I wanted to be for the rest of my son's life. There was a lot there to cope with in the early days.

Assessment

Jason attended the OZC for an assessment, where he told us that he was struggling to cope with the consequences of his strokes. He described physical difficulties including not being able to carry heavy weights, struggling to manage his balance, physical pain and excessive fatigue. He also reported feeling depressed, being unable to motivate himself, and having problems remembering to do things. He noted that he had difficulties getting the right words out and felt that his planning and keeping on task was 'not too bad but could be better'.

Cognitive assessment

Neuropsychological assessment revealed problems with attention, memory and executive functioning. Jason's scores indicated that he struggled to focus his attention, to keep things in mind and to remember things for the future (e.g. appointments). He also had difficulties in generating a plan of action, putting the plan in place and problem solving, particularly when a problem arose unexpectedly and he was required to think of a different solution.

Psychological assessment

Jason was clearly suffering with low self-esteem, depression and anxiety. Prior assessment had highlighted intrusive traumatic memories during his previous hospital stay, suggestive of post-traumatic stress disorder, but fortunately he now showed a significant decrease in the frequency and the impact of these intrusive thoughts. Jason told us that he often felt low and blamed himself for his strokes, noting that he always had a tendency to have high expectations of himself, and if he did not achieve these he was self-critical. He talked of feeling hopeless about his future and having low mood, but denied any suicidal ideation or intent. He experienced much frustration, mostly towards himself, as he felt like a failure since the strokes. He also noted that he had sleep problems, including insomnia, with negative thoughts often maintaining lack of sleep during the night.

Speech and language assessment

Jason had strengths in his social communication but did struggle to be assertive, resulting from his depleted confidence and low self-esteem. He also struggled to say things in the right order during conversations. Language assessment indicated no impairments aside from those requiring greater effort from memory and executive functioning skills.

Functional assessment

The Model of Human Occupation (MOHO; Kielhofner *et al.*, 1999) helped us to identify Jason's interests, values and perceived physical and cognitive skills for occupational participation, as well as his perception of his life roles, routines and environmental factors. Jason felt he was a failure as a worker and as a father. He was also unsure about his working skills. The assessment highlighted that Jason's most valued life roles were those of father, worker and hobbyist. It was not surprising, therefore, that he was feeling a negative shift in his sense of self as someone who previously achieved these roles and was always busy.

It was clear that the consequences of Jason's strokes had a serious impact on his life in many ways and that he wished to improve his quality of life for himself and his son, Joshua. We recommended that Jason return for rehabilitation and that he receive some prior motivational interviewing and counselling to prepare him for the programme. He found this particularly helpful and reported at the start of the programme that he was very clear about his goals and was 'raring to go!'

Rehabilitation

Jason attended the rehabilitation programme approximately five years after the strokes happened.

Goal 1: Jason will have a greater understanding of the impact of his strokes on his everyday life in order that he can develop strategies to manage these difficulties

Jason worked on this goal in both group and individual therapy sessions. He participated actively in the psycho-education groups; he was in fact often considered 'the rock' of the group by his peers who often sought advice from him, particularly in the Support Group. Jason shared strategies and tools with his peer group that he had developed in order to help himself prior to the programme. The 'therapeutic milieu' (Ben-Yishay, 1996) worked well for this particular group and for Jason specifically: it seemed to play a key role in enabling him to improve his confidence and self-esteem, which in turn played a role in helping him re-visit and re-connect with key aspects of his sense of identity.

By the end of the group phase, Jason had a clear formulation of the consequences of his stroke, which he shared with his family. As part of the UBI work, Jason set about deciding what project he would like to do to capture his understanding and his skills in a way that was meaningful to him. He chose to use his skills in carpentry and decided to create a 2D-image of a head and brain out of wood, demonstrating the different lobes in the brain. The outcome of this project is discussed in the next section.

Goal 2: Jason will develop strategies to manage the consequences of his strokes in order to be the best dad he can be to his son Joshua

Jason focused hard on his own specific goals during the second phase of the programme. His over-arching goal for rehabilitation, 'to be the best dad I can', was central to the process as he felt a real sense of discrepancy in achieving this since his strokes. He had described this role as key to his sense of identity in a personal constructs questionnaire developed at the OZC (see Gracey *et al.*, 2008 for details). At the start of the programme, as Jason felt he was an ineffective father to Joshua, most of the team members focused their interventions on this specific goal. In line with this, we asked Jason to test out strategies in functional situations using a behavioural experiment approach described later in this chapter. This phase of rehabilitation focused on one-to-one sessions with therapists and included sessions within the community.

Jason worked with a Rehabilitation Assistant to complete a portfolio explaining the consequences of his stroke in his own words. He reviewed his CT scans and did research on the type of strokes he had and the functional consequences linked to these. Jason also completed his 2D-brain project, which he presented at the Community Meeting. This project enabled Jason to test out strategies he had learned during rehabilitation as well as re-appraise old skills (such as carpentry). The woodwork project was a great success and Jason's sculpture was displayed proudly in the OZC main corridor (a photograph of this can be seen in Figure 10.1).

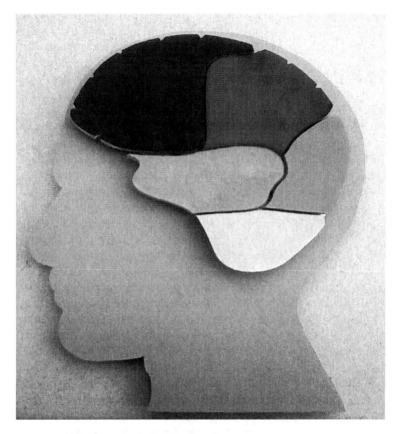

Figure 10.1 Jason's Understanding Brain Injury project: The 2D woodwork brain.

Jason worked with an Assistant Psychologist (under the supervision of a clinical psychologist) first to develop a shared understanding of his cognitive profile and then to develop strategies to compensate for his difficulties with executive functioning, including attention, goal neglect and prospective memory. We used a problem-solving approach adapted from Robertson's (1996) Goal Management Training (GMT). As part of this, Jason set text alerts on his phone to remind him to 'Stop–Think, am I on track?'. He also developed a personalised Goal Management Framework (GMF; based on GMT) to enable him to problem solve and make decisions. Jason's personalised GMF is shown in Figure 10.2.

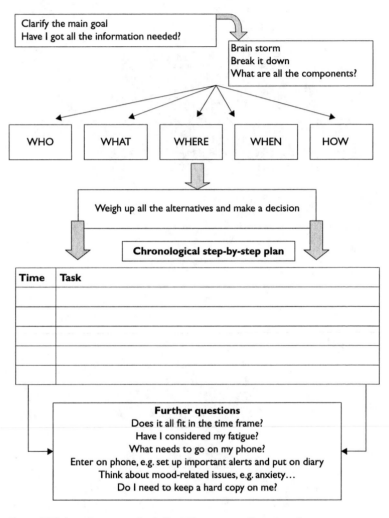

Clarify the main goal
Have I got all the information needed?

Brain storm
Break it down
What are all the components?

| WHO | WHAT | WHERE | WHEN | HOW |

Weigh up all the alternatives and make a decision

Chronological step-by-step plan

Time	Task

Further questions
Does it all fit in the time frame?
Have I considered my fatigue?
What needs to go on my phone?
Enter on phone, e.g. set up important alerts and put on diary
Think about mood-related issues, e.g. anxiety…
Do I need to keep a hard copy on me?

Figure 10.2 Jason's personalised Goal Management Framework.

After starting on the course I worked on my cognitive function, I learned all sorts of strategies with coping with my cognitive problems, the main ones for me are 'Stop–Think' and planning your day, week and month. This helped with not forgetting appointments etc.

Jason used his smart phone as his main memory and planning system since he was using it successfully prior to starting the programme. He integrated this well into his everyday life and needed no prompting to record prospective memory events and reminders on his smart phone. Jason applied these strategies to the problems he was experiencing in everyday situations and they are described in the occupational therapy section below.

Jason worked closely with his speech and language therapist to understand his communication difficulties in everyday life and learn strategies to manage them. The two key areas he chose were developing a strategy to verbalise information in the right order and developing assertiveness skills to deliver information in the best possible way. He was introduced to the '5 Ws and H' strategy (who, what, when, where, why and how) in order to organise how to verbalise information in a planned and ordered way.

The Community Meeting (the daily meeting of all staff and clients) was used as a vehicle to first test out this strategy. Jason used video feedback of himself in the Community Meeting to identify how this strategy had worked for him and what needed to be adjusted to make it more successful. He was then introduced to the Cornell method (adapted from Pauk & Owens, 2007) of note-taking to use key words to prompt information. He then role-played the use of the 5 Ws and H strategy alongside the note-taking prompts in a variety of social situations. A key part of this work involved enabling Jason to develop his assertiveness skills, which he had been introduced to in the Communication Group in the first phase of the programme. Feedback from Jason, and both staff and clients at the centre, indicated that he was more confident and assertive in his communication style by the end of the programme.

Jason attended individual psychotherapy sessions with a clinical psychologist each week. His initial goal for psychotherapy was to learn strategies to tackle his self-criticism, so that he would feel more confident and more content within himself. These sessions took a Compassion Focused Therapy (CFT; Gilbert, 2005, 2010a, 2010b) approach to tackling self-criticism, which we thought was underlying further symptoms of anxiety, low mood, low confidence and frustration, and to increase Jason's contentment within himself. A shared understanding of Jason's difficulties was formulated within the CFT framework. One of the key aspects of this was Jason's metaphor to describe the process of breaking the cycle or pattern of psychological difficulties by 'putting a spanner in the works'. He then did some self-guided reading on CFT and practised Compassionate Mind Training (CMT) strategies introduced in the Mood Group during the initial phase.

Jason began to realise that the consequences of his strokes were not his fault. It took some time for him to believe this, but through this process he began to break the cycle of beating himself up about the challenges he faced with his stroke. CMT techniques that Jason found most helpful in responding to his challenges to make him feel calmer included soothing rhythm breathing (a form of mindful breathing), compassionate 'safe place' imagery and continuously reminding himself that he had a tricky brain and tricky life, which were not his fault. He used a photographic cue on his mobile phone to aid compassionate safe place imagery in stressful situations alongside soothing breathing and encouragement to be compassionate and kind to himself and others by not rushing to problem solve when feeling overwhelmed. Jason incorporated strategies from his cognitive work into this, using his adapted 'Stop–Think' planning and problem-solving tool. He made strong gains during therapy, and the behavioural experiment approach allowed for excellent opportunities to test out his strategies for managing his mood.

After starting rehabilitation at Oliver Zangwill, I began to learn strategies to help with mood and cognitive function. I learned several different strategies really. I also learned that everybody has tricky brains at different levels. I learned that when I first started, what with being with five other clients – we've all got tricky brains, even in that small community. We all have different levels of tricky brains. One of the other things I learned about first was the three-circles model (from CFT), about our threat systems and our soothing systems. I learned that when the threat system kicks in it can really cause all sorts of issues like anxiety, but what I did learn was that by putting my 'spanner in the works' (that's my strategy that really helped to activate my 'soothing system'), I felt much better.

With my poor mood, I worked with Fi and we would work on Compassionate Mind Training exercises, which helped me so much I still use these exercises in my day-to-day routine, such as soothing breathing. With the breathing, I imagine myself on a surfboard. The sea would be initially very rough and choppy and through the soothing breathing the sea would become calmer, and so would I. I used the soothing breathing throughout the day really. I can be doing the soothing breathing while I'm actually talking to people now, before I couldn't, I had to really focus. That's really helped a lot.

At the end of the programme, questionnaire measures indicated that Jason had significant reductions in self-criticism, alongside increased ability to be compassionate and reassure himself, as well as reductions in frustration and a significant increase in self-esteem. At the end of

'Putting a spanner in the works'

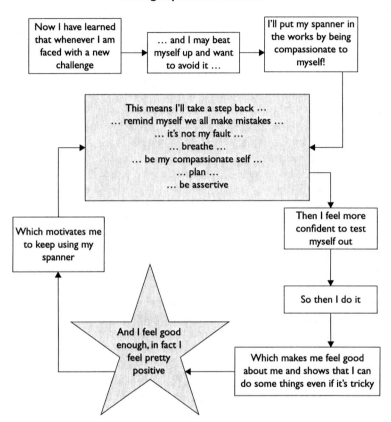

Figure 10.3 Jason's positive formulation.

psychotherapy, Jason developed a collaborative positive formulation, which can be seen in Figure 10.3.

Jason also suffered with insomnia and negative thoughts maintaining sleepless nights, which he wished to improve. While sleep difficulties are often under-assessed in this population, evidence is gathering for the importance of addressing sleep-related problems after acquired brain injury as they too have neuropsychological implications (Waters & Bucks, 2011). Therefore, additional separate sessions with a trainee clinical psychologist focused on psychological management of sleep difficulties. Jason began to learn about how worries and critical thoughts about his performance in tasks were affecting his arousal levels and consequently keeping him awake. In order to interrupt this pattern, Jason developed his skills in mindfulness that he previously learned in mood work. This enabled him to 'put a spanner in the works' as he described it, and reduced his worry and critical thoughts. This in turn led to an improvement in Jason's sleep, which had a number of positive benefits for his quality of life. For more details about this and psychological work see Ashworth, Clarke and Corfield (2012).

Prior to starting at Oliver Zangwill I had severe insomnia. After spending a lot of time with Alexis and Fi, I was able to control my sleep much more effectively. Instead of waking up three or four times a night four to five times a week, I now wake up once or twice – I monitor my sleep pattern on a daily basis. The strategy has had a great impact on my fatigue. Although I am on a lot of tablets, which can encourage fatigue, I'm now able to manage that so much better. I have also found out recently that I have very low oxygen levels in my blood, after having numerous tests at Papworth Hospital. I now have to sleep with a full face mask on while having a dose of oxygen fed into the system. It's improved my life so much now, with improved sleep.

The sleep work overlapped with occupational therapy, as Jason experienced debilitating levels of fatigue on a daily basis. He gained a clearer understanding of its impact and learned effective coping strategies including pacing, mindfulness and planning activities in advance. Jason also developed a system to consider how fatiguing or energising different activities: were using a points system so that each day he could think about how to balance activities depending on the amount of points used (an adaptation of the WeightWatchers approach).

As previously mentioned, Jason's main goal was 'to be the best dad I can be', therefore the strategies learned in all other sessions were put into practice in functional activities that he related to being a good father and which he would have completed with his son prior to the stroke. He did this work in individual sessions with his occupational therapist. One of Jason's key goals was to take Joshua to the Natural History Museum in London, but he did not feel confident to do this right away. Other goals included cooking for Joshua and taking him on holiday.

Therefore the team designed behavioural experiments (Bennett-Levy *et al.*, 2004) in the form of a graded hierarchy of activities for Jason to achieve these different goals. As is protocol with behavioural experiments, Jason made predictions about his perceived abilities, his emotional state and his fatigue levels for each planned activity. He also considered what cognitive, mood and communication strategies could support him in each activity and appraised how helpful (or unhelpful) they would be in a particular situation. A key ingredient of this approach was for Jason to reflect afterwards on these predictions and appraise the situation and strategies and his performance. During these experiments, Jason success-fully used cognitive strategies (e.g. Stop–Think and GMT, setting alerts and reminders on the phone), mood management tools (CMT and mind-fulness) and communication strategies (e.g. assertiveness). Through this process, Jason had a much greater sense of autonomy and felt less anxious, more confident and much more able to do activities through using strategies. He succeeded in taking Joshua to the National History Museum and even problem solved a number of unexpected situations that happened along the way.

The personal identity constructs questionnaire was re-visited throughout rehabilitation as a guide to assess whether Jason felt he was becoming 'the best dad I can be'. By the end of the rehabilitation programme, his response on this questionnaire indicated that he was much closer to reaching this goal.

Goal 3: Jason will develop a vocational action plan for moving forwards with work-related activity, will identify work-related skills, and will put together a realistic vocational action plan

With the continued use of the MOHO model as adapted at the OZC (Winson, Saez-Martin, Brentnall & Malley, 2012), Jason explored his vocational identity and began to think about what work he wished to pursue. He identified a number of possibilities including woodwork or carpentry and catering. However, he later ruled out catering using his GMT tool. Jason's vocational action plan involved continuing to look for work in woodwork and carpentry after the programme. This plan was also supported by his occupational psychologist at Job Centre Plus and by his Disability Employment Adviser (DEA).

Through the functional work, Jason increased his sense of efficacy in his role as father. Overall, his performance and satisfaction with occupa-tions was much improved by the end of the programme as rated by the Canadian Occupational Performance Measure (COPM) (Law *et al.*, 1990).

I think it's changed my life a hell of a lot now. From what it was just a year ago, I wasn't able to do any stuff like volunteering or college, whereas now I can do two days of volunteering and three days at college. I've got a busy, busy week.

Outcome

Overall, Jason made excellent progress during the rehabilitation programme and in the review period. He established excellent core knowledge of the consequences of his stroke and was able to develop specific strategies to manage these difficulties, leading to an improvement in his quality of life. Jason says that he is now enjoying the fruits of fatherhood with Joshua. From early on in rehabilitation, Jason appreciated the value of goal setting and this was apparent even after he finished the programme, as he has continued to use this approach in his daily life. Furthermore, Jason has also been a valuable contributor to educational days at OZC. He recently spoke to a group of health professionals about his experience of sleep and fatigue problems and described what had helped him in his recovery. He was the most popular speaker of the day!

My self-criticism isn't so bad now, don't get me wrong there is still a tiny bit there, but there is not so much as there was before. And also I don't tend to avoid things now, I tend to face them, I get on with them now. I found in the past if I avoid the problems, the issues become far worse than they were before. Now I have the right tools in my toolbox I feel I can carry on with my future.

Since I left Oliver Zangwill I have also completed three college courses: level 2 English Literacy, level 1 and 2 Mathematics, ECDL level 1 and 2. I am finding it hard to find an ideal vocation – I am currently volunteering at Oxfam in Peterborough, where I look after their website on a Tuesday and Thursday. I also socialise far more now than I did before, I currently meet up several times a week with family and friends. I feel the future is looking far better now I've had the help from Oliver Zangwill.

Chapter 11

Christine's story
One day I woke up and there I was![1]

Barbara A. Wilson and Christine

Christine, a divorced mother of four and grandmother, lived with her dog and cats and was devoted to her large family. At age 50, she developed tuberculous meningitis. For over two years she was mute, stuporous and barely more than minimally conscious. Then she started to recover. Although she remains in a wheelchair and has cognitive difficulties, she is now sociable, chatty and a different person from the one first assessed in 2010.

Introduction

Before I became ill, I lived in a two-bedroomed flat with one dog and three cats. We spent a lot of time decorating, me and the three girls. My ex-husband is a gypsy. He's got five brothers and five sisters. There's only me in my family and two step-brothers. My two sisters-in-law have two children each so it's quite a big family. One of my daughters has a little girl so I also have a grandchild.

I was very happy and happy-go-lucky before I became ill. I didn't care about anything and was always up for a joke. Me and the girls had lots of laughs. My Mum was the one who was steadier. She was the boss and she told us things straight. I speak to my Mum every day now. She phones up and we talk about everything. I like talking to her. She's a great support. I used to do hairdressing from home up until the time I became ill. I used to do everyone's hair.

What is tuberculous meningitis?

Tuberculous meningitis (TBM) is a bacterial infection of the meninges, the membranes surrounding the brain. It is one of the commonest forms of central nervous system damage in developing countries, particularly sub-Saharan Africa, but is also on the increase in the United Kingdom. Tuberculous meningitis is now a treatable disease, and recovery can be expected in over two-thirds of all cases. Not infrequently this takes place after periods of confusion lasting for months.

We include Christine here, as one of our survivors, because she made an unexpected improvement after an extremely long period of reduced awareness. Late-stage recovery long after a severe brain insult has occasionally been documented in patients with traumatic brain injury (Arts, van Dongen & Meulstee, 1988; Sarà et al., 2007; Sancisi et al., 2009), and in patients with Korsakoff's Syndrome (Victor, Adams & Collins 1989), but rarely, if ever, in conditions such as TBM.

Background of injury

Christine, herself, cannot remember this period of her life but her mother gave the following account:

It started in April 2008. Christine wasn't feeling well, she was nauseous and had lost a lot of weight. She went to the doctor and he thought it was anorexia. He referred her for a hospital appointment and we finally got an appointment for November, but by that time Christine was in a coma. We went back and forth to the doctor's. I knew things weren't right. She wouldn't let me go with her but her daughter went once or twice. In October Christine was really nauseous and weak and trembly. One Friday in October she went to bed, sick, hallucinating and with terrible headaches. She frightened the life out of us. She'd had TB before. She caught it from her partner but they hadn't picked that up at the doctor's.

We called an ambulance and she had a fall before the ambulance people came. They got the doctor out and they took her to hospital. She was kept in and one and a half days after she was admitted she went into a coma. This was still October (2008). They diagnosed tuberculous meningitis there. She was in intensive care but was then taken to a London hospital. I didn't know TB could jump like that. I'd grown up with TB, during the war it was rife, but I didn't know it could jump to the brain.

Christine was in a coma for six weeks and stayed in the London hospital for a lot longer than that. She was then moved to a hospital nearer home. A social worker there said the Raphael Medical Centre would be the best place for Christine and in June, I think it was, she moved to the Raphael. She was on TB medication for two years; it stopped while she was at the Raphael. For a long time her eyes were open but she wasn't talking and seemed to be comatose.

Christine was admitted to a hospital near her home in late November 2008 with a history of headache, altered consciousness and third nerve palsy. Early in December she was transferred to a London teaching hospital where she was diagnosed with TBM with secondary vasculitic infarction. A CT scan showed communicating hydrocephalus with ischaemic change. Hydrocephalus is frequently seen in patients with TBM (Garg, 2010). Christine was immediately started on therapy for TBM (Ethambutol, Pyrazinamide, Rifampicin, Isoniazide and Pyridoxine). This medication was gradually reduced and ceased completely in January 2010.

In late December 2008 Christine was transferred to a neuro-rehabilitation unit where a further CT scan was carried out in 2009 that showed a small increase in the size of the lateral ventricle and the third ventricle. Periventricular low attenuation was seen around the right lateral ventricle. There was no evidence of an intracranial bleed. So from the two CT scans it would appear that Christine had sustained an ischaemic right hemisphere stroke. Stroke is seen in up to 57% of TBM patients (Misra, Kalita & Maurya, 2011). An MRI scan carried out in January 2010 indicated 'moderately severe hydrocephalus (presumed communicating hydrocephalus related to TB meningitis). Unchanged since June 2009. No new abnormality'. In June 2009, Christine was transferred to the Raphael Medical Centre, where she received a combination of anthroposophic and conventional rehabilitation (Enteria & Florshutz, 2012).

Assessment

Christine was first seen for a neuropsychological assessment in January 2010, 15 months post-diagnosis. When first seen, she was awake and appeared to be calm, but she was unresponsive. She did not speak or make any sounds, and did not point to objects or words that were presented to her. It was decided to assess her on the Wessex Head Injury Matrix (WHIM; Shiel, Wilson, McLellan, Horn & Watson, 2000). This is an observational scale for people in reduced states of consciousness. On one occasion only, Christine was heard to say three words: 'Yes' and 'Not really'. People who are fully conscious and aware would, of course, pass all items on the WHIM. Christine was then observed for the following 11 months, during which time she remained almost mute except for the occasional word such as 'Yes'.

In January 2011, 26 months since she was diagnosed with TBM, Christine appeared to become fully conscious, and in February 2011 she was reassessed. When she came for testing, she appeared to be a different person from the almost non-responsive woman seen a year earlier. She was alert, talkative, friendly and cooperative. She was far too good for the WHIM now so we decided to administer four tests that she could probably participate in. These included a test of reading, a test of naming, The Severe Impairment Battery (Swihart, Boller, Saxton & McGonigle, 1993) and The Middlesex Elderly Assessment of Mental State (Golding, 1989). She had serious difficulty with reading and mild impairment of naming. Christine did not appear to have visual object agnosia. On the Severe Impairment Battery, Christine's score was again in the impaired range but she scored well, or reasonably well, in some sections, namely social interaction, attention, memory and language. Her overall score was low because she could not point, copy or gesture, so failed all items where she was required to move her hands such as writing her name, copying a square or demonstrating how she would use a cup. On the Middlesex Elderly Assessment of Mental State, she failed several subtests including orientation, arithmetic, comprehension, fluency and remembering pictures.

Christine did not have a motor disorder. She could move her hands when asked to point to body parts on herself and managed this without difficulty. She could demonstrate 'how to wave goodbye' and 'how to blow a kiss'. Yet when asked to show how she would use a cup or a spoon she failed to do the right thing, even when the cup and spoon were placed in front of her. When we said to her that she seemed to find it difficult to get her hands to do what she wanted, she said 'My hands are not cooperative with my brain'. This, we felt, showed insight. Although on other occasions she did not show insight and, indeed, seemed to be unaware of her situation. Thus, once she denied being in a wheelchair despite the fact that she was in a wheelchair at the time.

We wanted to know whether Christine could touch and point when engaged in other rehabilitation activities so observed her in Art Therapy and Music Therapy. In Art Therapy, she was seen to once point to a picture in a book with her right index finger. The art therapist put a brush in Christine's left hand (she was left-handed prior to her illness onset) and closed her hand around the brush. Initially, Christine rocked to and fro in her wheelchair and daubed paint on the paper as she rocked. Then she made some sweeps with the brush for a few seconds. She also appeared to smear some paint in one corner of the page when asked to paint buds. There was no other evidence of purposeful painting activity. Yet once again, some movements made by Christine looked perfectly normal: she pushed her glasses up from her nose several times and she held her hand to her mouth when she coughed. This confirmed our belief that she was not paralysed or weak.

Figure 11.1 Christine's painting of daffodils.

Christine was observed in Music Therapy two weeks later. She played the piano and we were very surprised to see that she used her right hand reasonably well, using most of her fingers. She also used her left hand (especially when her arm was positioned on a pillow), but not as well as the right hand. The difficulties with her left hand were likely due to a left hemiparesis (from a probable right hemisphere stroke). However, it was unclear why she had previously been unable to use her right hand to point to things in space. Christine was still recovering, however, and changing rapidly and from then on she started to reach out, point to, touch and hold things regularly. She was not always accurate though and when given a block-tapping task, she often failed to touch the correct block.

From then on, Christine seemed to go from strength to strength. For the next few months she was seen regularly. In September 2011 she scored a 100% score on the Severe Impairment Battery and showed normal naming. At this point, more traditional neuropsychological tests were administered. Christine was always willing to participate in the assessments and appeared to do the tests to the best of her ability.

From the results of these tests we concluded that prior to her illness Christine was probably functioning in the low-average range of ability. She had normal basic perceptual ability but impaired visuospatial functioning. She also appeared to have a degree of unilateral neglect, as suggested by her scores on the tests of neglect.

She showed serious impairments of speed of processing, attention, working memory, and memory. She also had difficulty with tasks involving reasoning and problem solving.

Although her memory score on the RBMT–3 was not good overall, she had acceptable scores on the verbal subtests. She was particularly impaired on the non-verbal/visual subtests, including face recognition and novel task learning. She had impaired recall of all periods of her life.

The most surprising thing about Christine, however, was the dramatic change she had made over the past two years. This change began more than two years after diagnosis and treatment for her TBM. When first seen in January 2010, she was almost totally mute and had a very low score on the WHIM. She appeared to be just beyond a minimally conscious state. In February 2011, she was a different person – being sociable, chatty and able to cooperate with the assessment. She then progressed from being assessed with tests for people with low awareness to being tested on more traditional neuropsychological measures.

Then everything changed about three years ago. I don't really remember anything. I know I had meningitis and TB but I don't remember becoming ill or being ill. I can't remember coming to Raphael Medical Centre but I remember being here and how I felt. I felt very angry. I didn't like being told what to do and when to do it!

People tell me I used to spend all my time sitting in a wheelchair and staring. I couldn't even talk or eat. But I don't remember any of it. It was like one day I woke up and there I was! I can't really remember when I became aware of things but it was at least a year before I knew where I was. It felt very strange to have lost so much time.

I was told I went to another hospital before I came here. I can't remember the previous hospital. I remember the physio here because physio used to hurt! I lost the use of my whole left side and still can't open my fingers. My foot is inverted and my Mum's in the process of getting me a new pair of shoes so I can have a calliper on it to make it easier to walk. Eating's got easier. Writing I'm working on. Reading I've got no problems with and I love reading. And I love talking!

I feel a bit lost and lonely stuck here away from Mum and Dad and the rest of the family. Sometimes I feel I don't belong.

Sometimes I feel frustrated because I can't do everything I used to do, like knitting, sewing or embroidery. I used to be able to write and it makes me frustrated at times that I can't do it easily now. I can use my left and right hands, though! I do art therapy and I love the art. I have some on my wall.

What can we learn from Christine's story?

Not only did Christine show more cognitive deficits than those patients reported in the paper by Williams and Smith (1954), her improvement is also unlike any of those cases. Christine's visuospatial and face recognition deficits are likely to be a result of the right hemisphere vascular changes identified by the CT scans. Observations and test results are consistent with generalised, bilateral, cerebral dysfunction, affecting frontal, temporal and parietal regions, with a greater degree of right- rather than left-hemisphere involvement.

Some studies have reported that TBM patients became worse after the introduction of anti-TB medication (Kumar, Prakash & Jha, 2006; Blackmore, Manning, Taylor & Wallis, 2008; Lima *et al.*, 2012) but none, as far as we know, describe the reverse situation, namely significant clinical improvement after the cessation of anti-TB medication.

Christine's story shows that late stage recovery is possible in patients with TBM, even after a long period of unresponsiveness. Christine has not made a full recovery. Her family noted changes in Christine's temperament, personality and self-care. For example, she now swears frequently, something she would never have done before her illness. She was described as previously being more reserved but is now bubbly and cheerful. She also pays less attention to personal hygiene or appearance compared to prior to her illness. She is still in a wheelchair and has significant cognitive problems but she is fully conscious, sociable and engages fully in life.

I think I've done absolutely brilliantly! My reading and writing have come on. I read better now than before I got ill! Talking and eating have also come on really well. It's time I woke up and started living!

I feel very hopeful about getting back my own home and life. I can't live in my flat now because it's unsuitable and has three flights of stairs. So I'm hoping and waiting for a bungalow to be found so I can be with my daughters. They're excited too. They can't wait for me to come home.

When I think about anything which feels different now, I feel more confident. I don't get as angry as I used to before I was ill. The girls say I speak my mind now, more than before. They say I don't take people's feelings into account as much and that I'm more outspoken. I know this is true. But I feel happy and am very hopeful for the future.

Note

1 A paper on Christine has been accepted for *Brain Injury* (Wilson, Hinchcliffe, Kapur, Tunnard & Florschutz, in press).

Chapter 12

Adrian's story
Dealing with potholes on the road to recovery

Fiona Ashworth and Adrian Wright

A young workaholic engineer with a devoted wife and children, Adrian had it all. That is, until a road traffic accident left him with massive orthopaedic and brain injuries and turned his life upside down. Adrian first came to the Oliver Zangwill Centre (OZC) for rehabilitation a year after his accident, with good results. But a few years later, a personal disaster brought him back for Round Two.

Introduction

I was a UNIX system engineer and I looked after Abbey National Bank's computer systems, the high-end ones. It was good because I was always given big projects and tasks to do. It was a good, high pressured, interesting job to do. I felt I was a good father, a good husband, but it was hard because I did on average about 90 hours a week, including overtime. I was definitely a workaholic. But I was a dad as well. I have two children, one boy and one girl, aged 6 and 8 (at the time of the injury). I was happily married. Generally I was the one working, and the wife looked after the kids and the house we owned. Then one day, while I was on my way home from work to pick up my son to take him for a hospital treatment as he had leukaemia, a van decided to hit me head on at that point.

Background of injury

Adrian was just 29 years old when he was involved in the road traffic accident. He suffered a severe traumatic brain injury (TBI) and additional orthopaedic and abdominal injuries. The accident also caused visual difficulties: he had a right homonymous hemianopia and he had loss of peripheral vision. Unfortunately, there was no documentation available regarding his Glasgow Coma score, although Adrian's wife later recalled that it was 'the lowest you can get'. The exact length of time that Adrian was in post-traumatic amnesia is unknown, although it was described as significant.

A CT scan of Adrian's brain on the day following the accident revealed 'a small right frontal contusion. No midline shift or mass effect is seen'. A further CT scan carried out one week later reported 'an area of haemorrhagic contusion in the right inferior frontal region. This causes some moderate mass effect with slight effacement of subarachnoid space overlying this region and perhaps of right ambient cistern'. Adrian had other extensive injuries including bilateral pneumohaemothoraces, multiple fractures and contusions and lacerations to his large bowel resulting in an ileostomy.

It wasn't until six weeks after that I can really recollect. I woke up, I wasn't able to speak and I had a whole load of metal holding my leg together. It was very scary. It was a real trauma but I really didn't know what was to come. After the first six months of SALT (speech and language therapy) and physio, I also got MRSA while I was in hospital. They were rehabilitating me as to what day it was, when it was, where I was? Until I could answer those they really were not going to release me. It sounds like prison, but they were not going to release me until I hit my targets. They were also monitoring the pressure in my brain. I thought it was just a bump. It was only on release that I saw the pictures of my brain and how the bruise had killed a bit, the right frontal lobe. I think they told me before but I don't remember it. I was wondering if I was too good working on my goals to be released and I think I was probably released too early. Looking back, I don't think I was really ready to join society. I mean I started to notice that I couldn't do simple things that kids could do. I would lose memory of what I was doing, e.g. going into a room to do something I could not remember what I was doing. And making wrong decisions, for example I did the wrong thing – when something happened I did the first thing that came to mind, I didn't think about it.

I wasn't able to go back to work. They kept my job open for me for a year and a half. I couldn't remember the last ten years of my life. When I was talking to my wife I was confused. I kept mixing up the holidays I had been on. I felt below worthless; it was as if everything I knew or could do had been taken away.

Assessment

Adrian's case manager referred him to the Oliver Zangwill Centre (OZC). It was just over a year after his accident when he came to OZC for assessment. He was seen by an interdisciplinary team of psychologists, an occupational therapist and a speech and language therapist.

Cognitive assessment

Adrian underwent a neuropsychological assessment that indicated areas of strengths as well as difficulties impacting on his everyday life. Difficulties included encoding and recall of verbal material, selectively focusing his attention visually and slowed speed of processing. Adrian also struggled on tests of executive functioning where structure was not provided and for tasks that required novel problem solving. Adrian tended to jump ahead without stopping and thinking on some of the tests.

Mood assessment

Adrian felt exhausted and frustrated with himself and his situation since returning home. He was worried about his family and their finances but was lacking in motivation. He felt depressed and anxious and had lost his confidence in himself. He noted sleep problems, a loss of interest in things and feelings of hopelessness about the future. The family was also struggling to cope. The children had noticed that Adrian was much more frustrated and cross and Adrian struggled with role changes since his wife had to take on many of the responsibilities that he had previously undertaken. His wife felt stressed and struggled to cope with the situation. Adrian felt as though he was no longer 'the husband or dad I used to be'.

Speech and language assessment

Cognitive difficulties affected Adrian's ability to interact with others. We noticed that he was tangential, often losing track of what he was saying. He felt he lacked social skills and tended to compensate by talking in an over-excited manner.

Functional assessment

Adrian struggled with activities of daily living, noting that he was more clumsy, needed prompting to do tasks, and often found that he needed support from his wife to do simple tasks such as making a sandwich. He particularly struggled with childcare activities; having lost his driving licence, he had to rely on his wife to transport the family. He also found it hard to focus on play activities with them. Adrian experienced significant fatigue, which affected his performance during the assessment, and of course it impacted on his ability to take part in his everyday life.

In summary, Adrian had a number of interacting cognitive, emotional and physical impairments as a result of the TBI that made it very difficult to continue with his life in the way he had prior to his injury. These types of difficulties were ideally suited for treatment within a holistic neuropsychological rehabilitation framework, and therefore it was recommended that Adrian return for rehabilitation.

I started seeing lots of specialists because of the accident. One of them said they thought there was a good place that could help me, so they (case manager) contacted you to see if you could help me. I remember I came for a one-day assessment. I was so down and so depressed, I thought 'no one can help me' – I thought they couldn't help me. Then I came back for a longer assessment. It was the first time I stayed on my own since the accident. Again I was so unable to receive help, but I was trying everything, by the end of it you said you could help me. But I still thought 'you can't'. I thought I was unhelpable.

Rehabilitation

Adrian attended the holistic neuropsychological rehabilitation programme with the goal of understanding the consequences of the TBI alongside developing strategies to cope with the resulting challenges. As with all rehabilitation programmes at the centre, Adrian worked with all members of the team to achieve his goals.

Adrian learned strategies to improve his planning and problem solving, including Goal Management Training (Robertson, 1996). He also learned strategies to manage his difficulties with verbal memory, although he had trouble remembering to initiate the use of strategy tools and needed prompting to use them as they were not 'automatic'. Psychological work focused on increasing Adrian's confidence using behavioural experiments (Bennett-Levy *et al.*, 2004) to challenge negative assumptions. Communication work also focused on developing Adrian's skills and confidence in social situations, using planning and preparation tools from cognitive rehabilitation sessions. Further work focused on improving his assertiveness skills. Adrian also developed a fatigue formulation and learned helpful coping responses to manage fatigue.

Since one of Adrian's main goals was to better understand his brain injury, he completed a UBI (Understanding Brain Injury) project with the help of his family. The purpose was to illustrate his journey through injury and rehabilitation and to flag up the important elements of his life, particularly his family. He wanted to work with wood as he related this to the brain because it was strong but could be easily damaged. He chose to create a large wooden cube with each side depicting one of the seasons of the year. The seasons were symbolic and each represented a time in Adrian's life. His children helped to decorate the box and he shared it with the team and his family at the end of the programme.

I decided to come for rehab. I think I was a difficult case because I was so shut-tered. I liked how you did it, having the four of us in and first teaching us about the brain – understanding which bits are working and which bits are not. I remember learning about the right frontal lobe and what it does, and I remember thinking 'ah, hmm, I see' and then I started to become more open to listening to the help offered.

The more we learned about the brain, the more things that hit me. I learned things where I thought 'ah, that's me, that's difficult for me'. Initially I thought 'hmm, that is bizarre' rather than thinking 'oh they know what they are talking about'. For me I needed the six months ... the poor psychologist .... I think it must have been hard for him because I kept thinking 'I don't have a mood problem' so it must have been hard to get past the shutters in the psychological sessions to work out how he could help me. But it's good he got there. The sessions really helped me with simple tasks.

The role of the right frontal lobe was explained to me, and I learned that if I 'stop and think' I could bypass that instant thought and then break it up into simple tasks. Basically doing what the right frontal lobe normally does in a more methodical way. It was very good at getting me to try things out – experiments – 'go try that out, let's see what happens'. When things began to start working, I became more receptive. Just implementing the. . . what was it. . . how to stop and think – I drew a picture of my wall, oh the GMF – can't remember what it stands for (Goal Management Framework). Yes my GMF diagram was, it was so person-alised, and I kept this piece of paper by me all the time. Not to start with, I only used it with big problems, but then I realised it could be used for any problem, even making a cup of coffee. Initially I thought 'don't be so silly, you don't need it to make a coffee', but when I started using it for that, it made me understand how it worked so well.

I was starting to do things and I was succeeding. At the time it felt good, but I was still dragging myself down until the end of it (rehab) about how I could do it a lot better before. I kept looking back to the past and comparing myself, how I could have done things better. But looking back now I might have been slightly glorifying my previous life, which was difficult to get back to. So once I was able to 'reset the zero' and stop looking backwards and comparing myself, I was able to start looking from 'now' rather than the past, I was amazed about what I could do. I would say to myself 'oh last week I couldn't do that, but now I can – I can do that. I thought I would never do that'.

My overall sense of the rehab, the outcome, was so very satisfying. For the first time since the TBI I was looking forwards, to trying things and being able to do things. My future – I was looking forward to doing things with my daughter, my son, and my wife. I went into the programme depressed and as if life was finished, waiting for death, but came out of it looking to the future, being better, being stronger.

Outcome and life after the programme

Adrian made significant progress during rehabilitation. His confidence increased and he developed the best tools to compensate for the difficulties he was experiencing as a result of the TBI. Due to the severity of the injury, he continued to need support after the programme. He was not able to return to work, but he still did some volunteer work. Adrian began to rebuild his life and, although he felt he was making good progress, he was struggling in the family context. This continued for the next three years.

In my opinion, I don't think my wife accepted me back as a husband. It seemed different, and it dragged me down a bit. I felt I was fighting to get better. But then my wife left me. Well, I had to move out. I don't think I was accepted for who I was. I felt I was succeeding by applying myself, but I don't think some of those around me felt the same. I thought here I am making significant progress, doing voluntary work, I also felt better in myself, feeling good about myself. But my wife leaving me – she hadn't accepted me back in her life properly. I think she thought I was going to die. She decided to divorce me under very difficult circumstances. It threw me back into depression, I felt I was useless, worthless and everything I did was rubbish. It was the first big hit since the programme that knocked me back. I was sat doing nothing, thinking 'life eeeh', which was bad. I started to believe that maybe the progress I made was luck, that I hadn't been able to do it. I felt everything about me was bad. I spent a lot of time arguing with myself as I believed what I was doing was good, but because the other part of me (what I called the Adrian bully) was saying I was rubbish, I was worthless, it took over. I felt everything that was happening was feeding the bully. I started to believe the bully in me.

I moved in with my sisters and thought I was ruining their lives too, so I moved out into a small two-bedroomed flat on my own. Unfortunately the Adrian bully got very strong then. Initiating anything was always difficult. I was trying to plan ahead but it would get over-ridden by the bully, which would say 'don't bother, you are not worth it, you won't be able to do it, don't even try'. I also didn't have the right support workers with me, which didn't really help either. I was also trying to see my children, but every access I had was good to some extent but I was always feeling like I was being put down. It was a difficult situation not to have the children living with me and that I had to ask for access. I was putting myself down a lot, believing all the negative things about myself. I spent a lot of time arguing with myself, but the Adrian bully was too strong to fight. The bully was so strong even if the milk went off I believed it was my fault (Adrian lost his sense of smell as a result of the TBI).

Round Two

Given his difficulties, Adrian's case manager realised he needed some more input to cope with this adverse life event. He could have gone to local services, but due to the difficult circumstances of Adrian's breakup with his wife, he found it very hard to trust health professionals. However, what he did feel was a strong sense of trust with staff at the OZC. He recognised that he needed help and he said he would like to try to get help from the centre again. Adrian returned to the OZC for an assessment. During this interview measures were taken of Adrian's mood state and his obvious self-criticism. It was evident that Adrian was severely depressed and experiencing some anxiety. He grappled with living alone and trying to cope with doing things he did not previously do in the home. He was also struggling to implement the strategies he had learned at the centre and was generally struggling to initiate and organise himself functionally.

Returning for further rehabilitation

At the end of the interview we decided that Adrian should return for psychological therapy alongside working with an occupational therapist to help him to be doing more. This combination of doing and meaning, which had previously helped Adrian, was identified as the means to move forward. Adrian identified his main goal as being able to lift his mood, reduce his self-criticism and have a nicer relationship with himself, and be more caring. The main goal was recorded as follows:

To find out who I am, how best to do things, and discover the 'Compassionate Adrian'.

The rehabilitation focused on the following:

- psychological therapy to support Adrian to adjust to the change in his circumstances and cope better with the strong emotions this had triggered;
- review of his existing coping strategies and development of new strategies for managing a range of activities that supported his sense of identity;
- training for his support workers to maintain the development and implementation of strategies specific to Adrian's needs.

Interdisciplinary rehabilitation consisted of 15 face-to-face sessions at the OZC, two sessions in Adrian's own home and a final review meeting held with the therapists, Adrian, his case manager and one support worker. Therapy consisted of sessions with a clinical psychologist and an occupational therapist on an individual basis and joint sessions to recap key learning points and agree independent work to be undertaken in between sessions to support new learning and generalisation of skills. Psychological input took a Compassion Focused Therapy approach (CFT) (Gilbert, 2005, 2010a, 2010b) to support Adrian towards the goal of becoming more compassionate towards himself. Therapy included a review of strategies introduced to Adrian during his previous rehabilitation programme at the OZC in addition to learning new strategies and skills. Adrian's support workers were involved and this proved invaluable in supporting the process of learning. They were able to help Adrian initiate skills and strategies in different contexts in between sessions. They were also able to modify the tools based on their shared understanding of Adrian's needs and our approaches. They shared information with other people in his support system where appropriate.

I started to make sense of my bully with the psychologist's help. We drew out a diagram of what was happening and what the function of my self-criticism was. I could see it clearly then, but it was still hard to see in the time when I was having a dark moment. It felt like the bullying voice was coming in from everywhere. I started to learn about this idea of being compassionate to myself – I was confident in you (OZC Team) from before, but the bully popped up and said 'there is no point'. It was fighting against the bully, I was open to it, but at the time I didn't believe it would work. I was open to trying it but the bully was not!

I started to learn to be more loving to myself. I have to say, the recordings (Compassionate Mind Training; CMT) were very important and necessary for me.

I started listening to them repeatedly – initially the calming ones (soothing rhythm breathing), the compassionate breathing which took me to a place where I was kind to myself. Then I started imagining myself being at my most kind, my most compassionate, what I then called 'Compassionate Adrian'. It seemed to start weakening the bully and strengthening the Compassionate Adrian. The more I practised it the stronger it got. Realising I am not alone helped; it's not just me that has these problems, others do too, life can be tricky, no one does everything perfect, and we all have hiccups that are not our fault. That was my Compassionate Adrian. But I did have a mental battlefield. Adrian bully had 98% of the territory and Compassionate Adrian only 2% but I was feeding Compassionate Adrian using the recordings, like meditation, and he began to get stronger and his territory became more, it was a good game of risk for me.

During this outpatient rehabilitation programme, Adrian demonstrated and reported use of old skills and strategies such as the GMF, fatigue management, weekly and daily planning sessions and internalising new skills such as CMT techniques including soothing rhythm breathing and compassionate self and imagery as well as identifying comfort zones in different domains in his life. Examples of skill application included the following:

- having a weekly review and planning ahead session with his support worker using a whiteboard to note forthcoming events as well as developing an IT-based system to support the planning and communication process;
- using 'STOP-THINK' and GMF before responding to situations and when making decisions, e.g. in interactions with his children and ex-wife;
- a better awareness of signs of fatigue and how to respond to these signs more effectively, such as changing the nature of the activity from mentally to physically effortful, taking breaks, altering plans, pre-empting and planning for tricky situations, being compassionate to himself;
- increased awareness in situ of the interactions between high levels of fatigue, low mood and behaviour;
- the importance of noting achievements and setting himself new goals, e.g. through use of 'comfort zones' diagrams in different domains of his life;
- use of CMT tools in responding to challenging situations, feelings and thoughts, e.g. high self-criticism;

- using a 'behavioural experiment' approach to check out if ideas about what may happen in a given situation actually occur, e.g. to test out strategies or perceptions about himself;
- having greater confidence in his 'positive parenting' approach following attendance at parenting classes, e.g. the development of 'house rules' with the children.

Outcome

At the end of the outpatient interdisciplinary therapy, Adrian and his therapists agreed that he had met the goals outlined. He reported that he felt more able to talk about 'normal things', rather than simply his injury, that he felt happier in himself overall, more comfortable in his own home and community and more confident in his own skills. This was evident to both his therapists and his support workers. He was also much more actively participating in a range of activities during the week, and had increased opportunities to interact with his peers. He had started helping out in the local village, as well as attending fitness classes and parenting classes and had even hosted a poker night at his house (an event he had previously attended at other people's houses but had never hosted himself). He made choices about what he wanted to do, i.e. what fitted with his own sense of identity. This progress was significant, particularly given the ongoing challenges Adrian was facing including medico-legal appointments, divorce and moving house.

Pre- and post-ratings were taken, as is standard in rehabilitation, and Adrian's ratings confirmed these reports of goal attainment. In particular, clinical questionnaires indicated a significant level of reduction in psychological distress as compared to the beginning of the therapy. Symptoms of both depression and anxiety had decreased. More specifically, Adrian's initial assessment had highlighted a coping style of criticising himself when things went wrong, leading to low mood and avoidance. Adrian then struggled to reassure himself that things would work out all right. The intervention of CFT enabled Adrian to build a new way of coping, that of being kind and compassionate to himself through the processing of CMT. CMT has enabled Adrian to respond to tricky and difficult situations or emotions in a way that leads to a sense of calmness, control and wellbeing and has reduced his self-criticism and tendency to avoid, as well as having increased his confidence.

I started doing more things myself. I also found that I was able to be more compassionate to myself, even towards the bully side of me. I decided that the bully side of me could come out when dangerous things might be about, to warn me, but the rest of the time, 98% of the time, I wanted to be Compassionate Adrian and I felt I was becoming him. It was amazing how much smaller he (the bully) got when I was being compassionate to him. I felt stronger in those moments. I felt stronger, more caring, more loving.

It was great to re-visit the GMF, I found that so helpful and I adapted it to incorporate the compassionate part of me too. As I practised it I found that it could be used, like before, for big and little decisions and planning. I also found that I could make decisions for myself, that I wasn't always trying to please everyone else, I was starting to think about what I wanted, what I thought was the right choice for me. The GMF just provided the foundation to work from.

It was evident that Adrian benefited from consistent support workers who have implemented therapeutic interventions and proactive case management. He also benefited from having structured time to practise using his strategies and reflect on the outcome of their use. As is standard, Adrian was provided with a template outlining his 'toolbox' of strategies, which he had developed collaboratively with his therapists. Adrian planned to share this with any new support workers and important persons in his support system.

I am now helping the vicar in the village, I have a lovely new home, I walk around the village every day and I can chat to people. I am also training for a marathon to raise money for head injury. I feel like I am now able to manage failure, I can more automatically find how to work with a problem. I feel much more confident in myself, I feel like I am getting to know myself better now. I also feel positive about the future, which is not a feeling I have had for a long time! It's been so good to have the support of my support workers too.

I found I was able to use the Stop–Think and GMF – they were working again, it was so good. Having the support workers was so helpful, having them there to remind me, to support me to use the tools when needed. But I also noticed that I was starting to think about using them without prompts from my support workers. I had a good example where I did this, I found myself in a tricky situation with picking up my kids, and it got fraught between my ex-wife and me. I was able to be compassionate and stand back and also think about how she might be distressed. I could stand in her shoes – it's not her fault or my fault. I reset my response and was calm and collected. It didn't ruin my day, as it would have done before. I was even using it with my support worker who was frustrated with the situation too; it was nice to help someone else! I found that I was using the tools automatically; it was becoming a part of me. I feel I have had a change of outlook on my life.

I thought being compassionate was alien, stupid to begin with. It was disgusting. It took a while, but I had to try very hard. Looking back, the bully was automatically filling the gap and he was so strong.

Practically, having the recordings (CMT) really helped me, as did re-visiting the GMF and having opportunities to practise using them with my therapists with real-life examples. The CMT recordings help plant the seed of being compassionate and then, after a few behavioural experiments, that really solidified it! It was a seed and now it feels like an oak tree!

For other survivors

I feel like it was really important to be open to it (rehab), no matter how negative your thoughts may be about it. For me, learning to be compassionate was so important and will be, to help me cope with the challenges to come, life doesn't stay the same and won't ever! It doesn't happen automatically, if you are looking for a quick fix for brain injury, there isn't one, just keep trying and open the mind, try step by step. I think the practice, keep practising was key so I would tell other people in my position to be open and practise, practise, practise!

For health professionals

This can happen to any of us, realising that we are no different from each other is important as often it could feel like somehow I was different, that I was less of a person. I think being able to trust the person, to have confidence in that person, is so important. I don't think I would have come back if I hadn't had such belief that the OZC team could help me again. I feel life is more meaningful for me now with being more compassionate to myself. If you are working with someone with a brain injury, be compassionate to him or her, it might shock him or her. They were compassionate to me, and that shocked me, it helped me, it might help other survivors.

Chapter 13

Lorraine's story

'I just want to be able to look after the bairns'[1]

Fiona Ashworth and Lorraine Allinson

Lorraine was a happy-go-lucky independent woman who enjoyed a good night out on the town with her best friend Andrea. She was always up for a laugh and enjoyed the single life. She was also a real 'mother hen' – her two children were always her priority and she doted on her two grandchildren and loved to spoil them. But a brain injury that led to post-traumatic stress disorder (PTSD) put everything in jeopardy.

Introduction

Lorraine is now a 55-year-old woman from Lincolnshire. Prior to her brain injury, she worked as a support worker for people with learning disabilities 25 hours a week, although she loved her job so much she would regularly work longer. She is divorced with two adult children, a daughter aged 22 and a son aged 19. She also has two grandsons aged 4 and 5 years; her daughter's children. Family, friends and the love of her job kept Lorraine young and happy.

Background of injury

Aged 50, Lorraine was involved in a road traffic accident as a front seat passenger. She was admitted to the Intensive Care Unit (ICU) at the Pilgrim Hospital, Lincolnshire, where her Glasgow Coma Scale on arrival was 15/15 and she was reported to be conscious. However, her period of post-traumatic amnesia was estimated to fall between 24 hours and 10 days, indicating a severe brain injury. Lorraine also suffered numerous orthopaedic, chest and abdominal injuries including punctured lungs, fractures of the jaw, humerus and spine and a ruptured spleen. Medical notes suggest that the primary mechanism of brain injury was hypoxaemia leading to brain hypoxia as a result of the damage to the lungs.

Lorraine's memory of the early days after the injury was that she had a number of strange experiences in hospital; health professionals had previously suggested that these may have been hallucinations due to medication she was on but she was adamant that they had happened and was therefore unwilling to accept this explanation, as it felt too real for her. After the acute phase of the brain injury, Lorraine did not receive any rehabilitation apart from some counselling sessions.

The symptoms I had relating to the PTSD were caused by the nightmares I had in ICU. The people that I was overprotective of were my two children and my grandsons. They all played a big part in the nightmares that I had in hospital. I had horrible thoughts about what I thought was going to happen to my family. I rang my children continuously and I never slept very well, as I was convinced that something terrible would happen to them. I would always think the worst scenarios; see them badly hurt or dead in my head. It has been the worst four years of my life.

After the injury, Lorraine had right-sided weakness of the leg and arm and walked with the aid of a stick. She struggled at home, and her son was concerned about her safety after some problems with cooking, so she went to live with him in his flat. Lorraine was also extremely anxious about the safety of her children and travelling in cars. Her daughter told us that Lorraine was often very tired and unable to do anything. She had not been able to return to work. She had problems with her memory such as forgetting conversations and misplacing objects. She also struggled to make decisions. She lacked confidence in her own ability to do anything. Lorraine had gone from being a fiercely independent sociable woman to being someone who completely depended on her family and her best friend. Those close to her said that the change was so significant it was hard to imagine she was the same person. Andrea said that where she had previously relied on Lorraine for support, this role had completely reversed. Lorraine's daughter also said that her mother used to be happy to babysit her children and had been a placid and gentle mother, but since the injury, she refused to babysit as she was terrified something bad would happen to the children under her care and she was constantly anxious and highly strung.

Assessment

After two years of struggling to recover from the brain injury, Lorraine was referred to the Oliver Zangwill Centre (OZC) for rehabilitation. The first stage of this process involved an in-depth assessment of the consequences of Lorraine's brain injury.

Cognitive assessment

Neuropsychological assessment highlighted difficulties with attention, specifically Lorraine's ability to sustain her attention as well as dual tasking. Assessment of memory highlighted problems with delayed verbal memory, immediate visual memory, topographical memory and prospective memory. Lorraine showed problems with aspects of executive functioning including inhibiting behaviours, understanding the consequences of her actions and decision-making.

Mood assessment

After the accident, Lorraine experienced increased anxiety about her family and her own safety, increased anger outbursts and social anxiety. She had begun to avoid social situations such as leaving the house and travelling in cars. She had also developed a dependence on having others around her at all times. Many of Lorraine's psychological difficulties were due to PTSD, which significantly affected her ability to function in her everyday life. Lorraine spoke about 'not feeling like herself' since her injury. Subjective changes in sense of self have been documented in the literature on brain injury (Gracey & Ownsworth, 2008). A personal constructs exercise was developed at OZC to try to capture this sense of change (Gracey et al., 2008). Lorraine's personal constructs highlighted that she felt less confident and less happy, did not know who she was and felt she did not understand herself or others.

Speech and language assessment

Lorraine did not have any severe speech or language impairments. However, the speech and language therapist observed cognitive communication difficulties such as going off track during conversations as well as repetition in conversation.

Functional assessment

Lorraine suffered significant physical pain and fatigue, which affected her ability to participate in her life in the way that she had done prior to the brain injury. Her fatigue was caused by the brain injury, but was exacerbated by anxiety (including hyper-vigilance) and pain. She walked with a stick due to physical injuries sustained in the accident and also to try to manage her pain. She struggled to do day-to-day tasks because of fatigue and pain.

In summary, Lorraine suffered with attention, memory and executive difficulties, severe anxiety, fatigue and physical limitations. As a result, she needed help with day-to-day tasks, was unable to work, had reduced social and leisure opportunities, experienced difficulties with travel and road crossings and was unable to look after her grandchildren independently.

Rehabilitation

Before I came to OZC I was in a bad way. What helped me about coming to the centre was being able to understand why I was the way I was after the accident. I couldn't get my head around it before.

Lorraine was highly motivated to return for the rehabilitation programme. Lorraine wanted to understand what was wrong with her as she could not make sense of the consequences of her injury. She also very clearly wanted to stop feeling so fearful and anxious so that she could get back to being 'grandma' to her grandsons. She also hoped to feel a greater balance in her relationship with Andrea, as she felt she had come to rely too much on her. She wanted to go back to being 'the old Lol' who was independent, happy go lucky and calm, but recognised that she might not be able to be exactly as she was before. Although work was not a high priority for her, she still wished to find out what work-related skills she retained so that she could explore work opportunities should she wish to in the future.

Together, Lorraine and her team set her goals for rehabilitation, initially focusing on increasing her awareness and understanding of the consequences of her brain injury more clearly, followed by helping her to develop and apply strategies to find ways around the difficulties with the brain injury.

Goal 1: Lorraine and her family will develop an understanding of the cognitive, communication, mood and functional consequences of her injury

In the intensive phase, Lorraine was encouraged to understand the consequences of her brain injury through a number of parallel processes. She attended the understanding brain injury (UBI) groups including Mood, Cognitive and Communication Groups to learn generally about the consequences of her injury with three peers who had also experienced acquired brain injuries. Participating in a group offered Lorraine and the other clients the unique opportunity to share experiences, learn from each other and support each other. In addition, Lorraine saw individual therapists to piece together each of these areas (mood, cognition and communication) and learn how they specifically affected her. Furthermore, this work was all drawn together in a one-to-one UBI session capturing an overall shared understanding of the difficulties Lorraine experienced in the form of a portfolio. In this session, Lorraine explored in more detail how different areas of her brain and body were injured during the accident, exploring time spent in hospital and investigating unfamiliar words that had been used in reports describing her injury. In the integration phase, the focus of Lorraine's UBI portfolio work shifted to compiling a strategy table enabling her to document all the strategies she learned in the different sessions over the course of the programme. Alongside her UBI work, Lorraine wrote about her experience and rehabilitation of the PTSD that she had suffered. These three separate pieces of work were brought together in a folder to make her UBI project, entitled 'Lorraine's Journey'. Lorraine's story in this chapter is excerpted from this project.

Lorraine attended the Support Group with her peers, a group that focused on psychological processes aimed at clients giving and receiving support (see Wilson, Gracey, Evans & Bateman, 2009 for more details about the groups). Lorraine was highly motivated during rehabilitation. She was an active and welcome member of the group and would often offer helpful and kind advice to her peers. She was productive and would always complete 'homework' assignments such as researching concepts about which she was unsure. At the end of the initial phase she had a good understanding of the consequences of her injury as well as an understanding of the types of interventions and strategies that she would try in the integration phase. Family support and education were also provided; Lorraine's daughter and son, Sarah and Jonny, and Andrea attended a UBI Day for relatives and friends as well as individual sessions with the psychologist to help them to understand the consequences of the injury and share their own stories of the impact of Lorraine's injury on them.

In the second phase of the programme, Lorraine and her team set clear rehabilitation goals.

Goal 2: Lorraine will learn and apply cognitive strategies to compensate for her cognitive challenges

Armed with a greater understanding of her cognitive difficulties, Lorraine wanted to develop strategies to use regularly to reduce the impact of her difficulties on the tasks she wanted to achieve. Most importantly, she wanted to better remember what she had read. When she read a chapter, she would forget what happened and have to start again. As a result, she had stopped reading books since her injury, something that she had previously particularly enjoyed. We used the analogy of a 'filing cabinet' to explore and represent the different components of memory and enable Lorraine to develop an understanding that each part of the memory process can be differentially affected by injury. She then explored and identified situations in which her retrieval of memories improved or deteriorated. Lorraine noted that she was more likely to remember to do something if she had written it in her Filofax (see goal on memory and planning system). She then tried noting down a few key points at the end of each chapter in order to avoid having to re-read sections of the book. She was delighted at being able to 'pick up where I left off'.

Lorraine wanted strategies to help retrieve and recall past events. We taught her to ask for cues about an event, which often helped her retrieve information about it.

Like many people with acquired brain injury, Lorraine had difficulties with dual tasking, or doing two things at once (Posner & Peterson, 1990). These difficulties were identified on the Test of Everyday Attention (Robertson, Ward, Ridgeway & Nimmo-Smith, 1994). Lorraine herself noted that while she felt confident selectively focusing her attention and reducing distractions so that she could complete one task, there were often situations in which she was required to concentrate on more than one thing at a time. For example, her walking deteriorated (deviating to the right) when she was simultaneously holding a conversation. Lorraine completed the Divided Attention Questionnaire (Bateman, Greenfield, Evans & Wilson, 2007), a self-rating of difficulties experienced when dividing attention. Scores indicated that Lorraine experienced the highest frequency of difficulties with: stopping an activity to talk; walking deteriorating when talking at the same time; and following a conversation when several people talk simultaneously.

We worked on improving Lorraine's dual-tasking ability using an evidence-based approach to training (Evans, Greenfield, Wilson & Bateman, 2009). The training focused on practising tasks that comprise both a motor and a cognitive component. In order to generalise these skills Lorraine identified specific functional situations that required the ability to effectively dual task, such as 'looking after the bairns'. On finishing the training, she completed the divided attention questionnaire again, and scores indicated a significant improvement in her ability to dual task. She also reported some improvement in her ability to walk and talk.

Occupational therapy sessions primarily focused on difficulties with executive functioning such as goal neglect and prospective memory. Lorraine learned two new internal cognitive strategies, the 'mental blackboard' (keeping things we intend to do in mind by writing on a mental blackboard) and making associations. She also learned adapted forms of goal management training (Robertson, 1996), using 'Stop–Think' to encourage her to reduce her compulsive buying. Lorraine reported that each time she thought of buying something while she was out shopping she would use Stop–Think and ask herself, 'Do I really need it?' An excerpt from Lorraine's UBI cognitive strategy table can be found in Table 13.1.

In the remaining cognitive sessions, Lorraine reflected that she had become much more aware of her cognitive difficulties and how to deal with them. For example, she addressed her difficulties with topographical orientation by developing the strategy of self-talk – specifically noticing and telling herself important recognisable landmarks that she could find again. Consequently, to increase her understanding of the different levels of awareness, Lorraine developed her own model, based on Crosson *et al.*'s (1989) model of awareness. She mapped her own experiences on to these levels, which increased the overall level of awareness that she reported feeling.

Goal 3: Lorraine will learn how to keep on track in conversations

Early on, Lorraine realised that she was repetitive in speech during conversations and struggled to keep up with the chatting around her. She learned to use clarification when she was talking to avoid repetition and to help her stay on track.

Lorraine's PTSD also led her to avoid social situations, which prevented her from taking part in social activities and meant she had fewer opportunities to test out strategies in conversations. We used the framework of behavioural experiments (Bennett-Levy *et al.*, 2004) to encourage Lorraine to predict her success using strategies in social

Table 13.1 Excerpt from Lorraine's cognitive strategy table

Cognitive Consequences I have problems with. . . .	This means that . . .	The strategy I can use to support me with this is . . .
Dual tasking	I have difficulty doing two jobs at once, e.g. sewing and cooking	Dual-task training I also try to concentrate on one job at a time
Memory (autobiographical)	I have difficulty remembering past events	I ask for cues about the event I cannot remember
Memory (prospective)	I forget important appointments and what my finances are	Filofax Mental blackboard Associations
Memory (topographical)	Navigating around unfamiliar places	Self talk. I notice and tell myself important recognisable landmarks that I will find again
Compulsive buying (making decisions)	I buy things I don't need or buy more than I need	Stop–Think Self talk. Asking myself 'Do I really need it?'

situations and then reflect on the experience. She adopted a number of strategies, including taking a rest prior to going out and using clarification in conversation. She began to report feeling 'more like my old self'. Lorraine's confidence in communicating in social situations increased so much that she felt she no longer needed communication sessions, and we agreed!

Goal 4: Lorraine will learn how to manage her fatigue to conserve her daily energy

Lorraine told us that fatigue impacted greatly on her ability to do her everyday activities. We gave her the 'Managing Fatigue after Brain Injury' booklet published by Headway (Cooper & Malley, 2008) and having read this, she had a better understanding of why she felt fatigued.

She and her occupational therapist (OT) then developed an individual formulation of her fatigue based on her learning about the factors that made her vulnerable to experiencing it. She learned which activities were more likely to be significant triggers and how she could monitor fatigue by noticing how she was feeling.

Lorraine found that many of the strategies and skills she developed during the programme enabled her to manage tasks more effectively and use her available physical and cognitive resources more efficiently. By the end of the programme, she used fatigue management strategies, including taking a rest before she went out for social activities in the evening, prioritising activities and pacing herself each day. However, given that her fatigue was neurologically based, there were times when she still suffered with severe fatigue that impacted on her cognitive abilities and was also exacerbated by pain. Despite this, Lorraine coped better with day-to-day demands when using the strategies, and overall she participated much more frequently in her desired pursuits compared with her participation levels prior to the programme.

Goal 5: Lorraine will reduce her anxiety and safety behaviours through actively taking part in cognitive-behavioural treatment of PTSD

Lorraine developed a shared understanding of her significant symptoms of PTSD with her psychologist. The two of them collaborated to develop a cognitive-behavioural intervention based on a cognitive model of PTSD (Ehlers & Clark, 2000). The intensive phase primarily focused on psycho-education about the nature of PTSD. During the integration phase, Lorraine focused on PTSD treatment including:

- using behavioural experiments to break the maintenance cycles of unhelpful behaviours (e.g. phoning her son and daughter excessively);
- re-living the traumatic memories and experiences in order to do cognitive re-structuring work;
- alongside the re-living work, planning a hospital visit once the cognitive re-structuring had been done in order to reinforce the understanding that the nightmares and hallucinations were not reality.

As is recommended by the National Institute for Clinical Excellence guidelines for the treatment of PTSD (NICE, 2005), we considered it important to involve the family in treatment. Both Sarah and Jonny agreed to participate in the process. They gained a better understanding of the impact of the PTSD on Lorraine and on themselves as well as learning to support her with the work. For example, we set up and discussed PTSD-related behavioural experiments jointly with Lorraine and her children. As time went on, Lorraine took on the job of liaising with Sarah and Jonny herself and this experience built her sense of autonomy. These experiments involved situations or activities that Lorraine had previously taken part in prior to the accident and subsequent PTSD, but which she now found too anxiety provoking to do (some of this work overlapped with cognitive communication work). Although anxious, Lorraine was highly motivated and completed all the behavioural experiments set. These included reducing the 20 plus phone calls a day to her children to only once or twice a day, walking to the shops on her own, crossing a busy road on her own, babysitting the grandchildren and taking the grandchildren to the shops. Lorraine also completed additional experiments with support from Andrea.

With regard to the second point outlined above, Lorraine attended extended cognitive-behavioural therapy (CBT) sessions in which she talked through her traumatic experiences, including the hallucinations and nightmares from hospital, and worked on changing the nature of these traumatic memories through exposure and re-processing. The CBT work also linked to her UBI project, which involved collecting information about her injury and hospital stay. The aim was to help Lorraine to safely retrieve emotionally overwhelming thoughts and memories about the hallucinations and nightmares during her hospital stay and to process these experiences to allow her to rationalise what was 'real' versus hallucinations and nightmares. This understanding of reality then became part of her ongoing autobiographical memories about her past experiences. Although it was emotionally difficult, Lorraine engaged in this work to her full potential. As was predicted, and is typical of this kind of work, there was an initial increase in symptoms before we started the work. However, they began to subside through the intervention process and Lorraine began to experience gains from the exposure and re-living work.

Lorraine visited the Intensive Care Unit (ICU) at the hospital where she was hospitalised after the accident in order to help with processing the trauma memories of the hallucinations and nightmares. This visit was very powerful; Lorraine met with her consultant neurologist who answered many of her questions about the traumatic memories from hospital. She was also able to see the layout of the ward, enabling her to re-appraise fragmented and traumatic hallucinations and realise that they were in fact hallucinations and not a part of reality, thus putting the memories into a better and less traumatic order. Lorraine's daughter, Sarah, had also been traumatically affected when visiting her mother in the ICU. She went with her on this hospital visit and afterwards the two of them had a reflective discussion that allowed them both to 'store' the traumatic memories and put them into the past.

Fi, at the centre, explained about the PTSD. Everything I was told about the PTSD work rang true. When I relived the nightmares at the time, it was torture, but I am pleased as I feel and look like a different person and I don't continuously ring my children. I still ring them every day, but not every hour like I used to do. I was at my daughter's on Wednesday and I took my two grandsons to the shop on my own. I was a bit dubious at first but they understand my problem so they both held my hand and it went very well. My daughter's partner's nephew turned 18, so I looked after the boys while they were out for a meal. They were in bed asleep when they went out, but I wasn't checking them as much as I would have done before. In fact I'd probably just have sat on the end of their beds until they came back from dinner!

I feel like a different person now. I am not on high alert 24/7 like I was before I knew what the PTSD was. We (Fi and I) went over everything that had happened. I am really happy that I found out about it and also I visited the ICU, which was arranged by Fi, as everything I thought was there from the nightmares wasn't there. I am just so pleased because I don't think I could have gone on much longer as I was. That in itself was a nightmare, and the not knowing why I was like the way I was, was awful. At one time I thought I was 'going round the bend' but now I've come out the other side and I can't thank them enough for getting me back to how I used to be. I'm feeling much more like the old Lol!

At the end of the intervention, Lorraine had made significant gains. She showed greatly reduced levels of PTSD symptoms on formal self-rating scales as well as subjective rating scales. She is much less likely to react as if under threat (e.g. anxiously, fearfully shouting) and is calmer in potentially difficult situations. Because it is known that individuals who have experienced PTSD may continue to be vulnerable to reactivation of symptoms in the future, a relapse prevention plan was set with Lorraine and communicated in a report to her doctor.

Now I don't think that bad things are always going to happen. I think more sensibly now if I can't get in touch with my children. I went to my grandsons' sports day and I watched them in the races. Before, I wouldn't have been able to go, I would have thought that they would have fallen and knocked themselves out, or broken their leg or arms or worse, died. I'm enjoying the times I spend with my children and grandchildren now, before I always thought that something terrible would always happen to them.

Goal 6: Lorraine will develop a memory and planning system to support her with budgeting and daily activities

Lorraine's functional sessions offered the opportunity to identify daily activities, including chores and leisure activities in which she could test out her strategies using behavioural experiments to reflect on the process and learn what worked best for her. Lorraine worked with her OT to develop systems and strategies for managing daily living tasks, including shopping, budgeting, planning, personal care and community mobility. During the intensive phase, Lorraine had identified difficulties with her current memory and planning system, and decided to trial a Filofax as an alternative. She was very successful and used her Filofax to manage weekly appointments and prospective tasks, including shopping lists. Lorraine developed an income and expenditure system to manage her budget that proved successful and worked well with her decision-making strategy to 'Stop–Think – do I really need it?' when she went shopping.

Lorraine achieved her goals of participating in leisure activities she previously enjoyed, including taking the grandchildren out independently, socialising with friends and crocheting. These goals were achieved through the integration of functional, mood and communication strategies; this integration of disciplines is a hallmark of holistic neuropsychological rehabilitation.

Goal 7: Lorraine will identify her work-related skills and develop a realistic vocational action plan

Lorraine and her OT explored potential voluntary work opportunities. They carried out a task analysis to consider what skills and strategies she had and may need to develop in order to undertake voluntary work. Lorraine secured a voluntary placement with an old-age home, where she spent a number of sessions and reflected on her skills and needs for future work. Lorraine also identified clear limitations to work, including her pain and fatigue levels and difficulties with managing her attention. She considered the strategies she would need to manage these difficulties. Lorraine developed a clear vocational action plan for the future, setting goals with the support of her case manager.

From a functional perspective, Lorraine achieved the goals set for the rehabilitation programme. Her accomplishments were reflected in her satisfaction and performance ratings on the Canadian Occupational Performance Measure (Law *et al.*, 1990).

Outcome

Overall, Lorraine made excellent progress during rehabilitation and she achieved her goals. It was clear from discussions with Andrea, Sarah and Jonny that they were very pleased with the progress she had made. Lorraine completed the Personal Constructs exercise again at the end of the programme, and results indicated that she felt more confident, happier and better understood by others, and she had a better understanding of her own feelings. Since leaving the programme, Lorraine has not returned to paid work, but she has been able to support her daughter, Sarah, with her two boys and the recent arrival of a new baby girl. Lorraine reported that she is very happy that she is able to do this now and says that although she still suffers with some occasional anxiety, it does not prevent her from doing the things she wants to do on a daily basis. Lorraine highlighted the ongoing challenges of pain and fatigue as preventing return to work.

I will continue the work now; I have set myself some goals. I took my grandchildren to the shops like I said above, and looked after them. The next thing is I'd like to take them out for the day in the school holidays. I never want to go back to how I was before I found out I had PTSD. My daughter, Sarah, is having a baby in October, I want to be able to feed the baby with a bottle. Before, I would have thought she would have choked. I never want to be how I was before in the last four years. I am thinking positively now. Before, it was all negative and the worst things that could happen. Now I am looking forward to the things I can do with my children and grandchildren and having a life again!

I am a lot better than I was before and I can deal with things a lot better. I also find that I can concentrate better on what I am doing. I only do one job at a time instead of getting waylaid and not getting anything done. I don't know how to really put it into words, but all I can say is that if I hadn't have come to the centre I would still have been going around in circles and never getting anything done or just constantly worrying about what was going to happen to my family (always the worst scenario ever). I still look after my family, my children and their bairns and sometimes I worry about them but not even half as much or a quarter as much as I used to.

Note

1 'Bairns' is a Scottish term for children.

Chapter 14

Mark's story
The 1,000-foot fall guy

Barbara A. Wilson and Mark Palmer

*Mark was in his early thirties and was a very successful international prop-
erty underwriter for a large insurance company. While on a mountain biking
holiday in Switzerland, he fell 1,000 feet down a mountain, sustaining a severe
traumatic brain injury. Following rehabilitation, Mark was able to return to
his previous post and has remained in employment ever since. He is now
married with two daughters.*

Introduction

*Before my brain injury, I think that I was a pretty level-headed guy, mostly single,
very motivated towards success at work and the trappings that entailed, maybe a
little egocentric.*

Background of injury

*On 2 September 1997 I had a 'tumble' whilst riding the Tour de Mont Blanc on a
pedal cycle and fell just over 1,000 feet down the Col Ferret. I was treated in
Switzerland where I had operations to relieve the intracranial pressure on my brain
and unfortunately also developed meningitis and septicaemia during recovery.*

Mark was airlifted to a specialist hospital in Switzerland where he was in
a coma for a week, and then experienced post traumatic amnesia (PTA)
for a further week. A CT scan showed diffuse axonal injury, oedema,
small deep midline haemorrhages and a subdural haematoma. The
haematoma was evacuated via a burr hole. He had a tracheostomy tube
in place for ten days.

*My attention and short-term memory were affected, as well as my ability to plan
ahead. Initially, I had trouble with my balance and obviously thence mobility, but I*

started walking again after I returned to the National Hospital in London. I've subsequently had a hip replacement as I developed osteonecrosis, which I understand was a result of my injuries and drug intake during my time in a coma.

Mark was transferred to London for acute rehabilitation. At this time he was ataxic and agitated and needed two people to help him stand from a sitting position. Although a good physical recovery was made, Mark remained with considerable cognitive problems.

From the National Hospital I went to the Devonshire Hospital in Marylebone where my clinical psychologist (the late Jolanta Ossetin) was keen for me to attend the Oliver Zangwill Centre for rehabilitation. I attended both one-day and week-long trial sessions before starting there as a full-time client (but staying in a guest house in Ely) for a year.

It was at the Devonshire Hospital in Marylebone where my first memories post-crash are from, and those are in cognitive sessions with the late Jolanta Ossetin. I felt at the time that Jolanta was being unduly tough with me – she was a real stickler for getting me to complete things entirely correctly – she really gave me no quarter. In fact, she told me to prepare myself for the fact that not only might I not be able to return to the job that I previously held, but that because of my disabilities I might not be able to hold down any form of gainful employment at all. Maybe she said these things because they were true at that stage of my recovery, but I like to think that she was just 'spurring' me on to succeed. Whatever her reason, it worked, and she is one of the cornerstones of my recovery. I continued to stay in touch with Jolanta long after I returned to work, also attending some of her piano performances, but very importantly invited her and her daughter to my wedding in 2008 where I was able to thank her personally in my wedding speech. It is with great regret that Jolanta is no longer with us, but I was very honoured to speak at her memorial service where I could tell everyone just how influential she had been in my life and how much poorer it would've been, and that I certainly wouldn't have been able to attain what I have to date without her involvement.

Aside from Jolanta, my first memory post-crash with regard to the Devonshire was that it was the first place where my family, friends and work acquaintances could come and visit me. I understand from an old colleague that she had to arrange a list each evening for the two and a half months that I was in that hospital for people to come and visit me. I began speech therapy, as well as some physical exercise in the gym there each day, along with many other cognitive and related sessions.

Dr Greenwood and Jolanta had a great struggle with my local authority to get funding for the Oliver Zangwill Centre but I'm so glad that they did as if I'd gone back into my previous job at that time (post the Devonshire Hospital), my career would've been over as I was nowhere near ready enough (as Jolanta had said) to go back into that (if any) occupation at all. I really wasn't aware of my disabilities and that would've given me an 'unemployable' tag in my market.

Assessment

Nine months after his accident, Mark was admitted to the Oliver Zangwill Centre (OZC) for neuropsychological rehabilitation. We were asked to help with his memory, attention and planning problems. He was described as lacking initiative compared to his pre-morbid personality and, although he had some insight into his difficulties, he did not appreciate the nature and extent of his memory problems or the potential impact of such impairments on his work. He said he had difficulty 'time-stamping' his memories. Because Mark had been assessed numerous times before coming to the OZC, he was given only a short neuropsychological assessment at the centre. He scored in the average range on a general intelligence test and in the above average range on a measure of pre-injury functioning. On memory tests his performance was poor, and on one well-known memory test, he scored in the bottom one per cent compared to the general population. In addition to his memory difficulties, Mark had some mild executive deficits causing him to have problems with planning and problem solving.

I guess that post the Devonshire Hospital (December 1997) I really just wanted to get back to work as all the friends and colleagues that had visited me kept saying that I was missed and just when was I coming back? I was still receiving a (reduced) payment each month from the permanent health insurance that I had in place through my employer but I wanted to get back to earning my old salary. I had also been given a company car in 1997, so I wanted to get back to that lifestyle. I thought that I needed someone to say that I was OK to return to work then my company would take me back on again full time. I thought that person would be at the Oliver Zangwill Centre and I was slightly perturbed that I had to go back for the two-week assessment after the one-day visit. I thought that the people at the centre would see that although I wasn't 100%, I was still good enough. How wrong I was! I remember being in floods of tears in a session with Jonathan Evans when he showed me that what my brain was and wasn't telling me just wasn't consistent and true.

Rehabilitation

Mark entered the holistic rehabilitation programme. With the rehabilitation team, Mark set the following specific goals for his programme.

Goal 1: To develop an awareness of his strengths and weaknesses in a written form consistent with his neuropsychological profile and describe how any problems would impact on domestic, social and work situations

To achieve this goal, Mark engaged in a programme that consisted of group work (e.g. *Understanding Brain Injury Group, Memory Group, Planning/Problem Solving Group*) and work with individual team members. There were many elements in Mark's programme, and one of the most critical was helping him cope with memory difficulties. His insight into these problems was achieved by education about the nature of memory and the problems that may exist after brain injury (through *Understanding Brain Injury Group* and *Memory Group*). He was given feedback from the result of standardised assessments. He was asked and prompted to keep a diary of memory errors. These were monitored. He was asked to consider his work role and to identify the demands on memory that are made as part of his work. He made good progress in appreciating his cognitive difficulties, particularly his memory problems. The work that he did in identifying potential consequences of his memory problems on his work situation enabled him to develop strategies to help him minimise the potential impact.

Mark developed better insight into his difficulties, which had a 'down-side' in that he began to feel low as he became less confident that he would be able to return to work. However, the rehabilitation team supported him in developing a set of strategies designed to compensate for the problems. He adopted these strategies successfully and started to use a large diary for appointments and 'things to do'. He began to use a computer 'contacts' card system for recording relevant information about brokers who came to him with business to ensure that he was up to date with relevant information such as how many children they had, dates of their birthdays and so forth. This was to ensure effective personal communication, an essential part of Mark's work. He also learned to use mnemonic strategies for remembering people's names and other information.

This was another cornerstone of my recovery as being made fully aware of my disabilities I could then work on strategies for compensating the said deficiencies to overcome them using internal as well as external strategies. To give an example of the use of an internal strategy that I still use to this day, the phone number for the Oliver Zangwill Centre was so ingrained into me during my time there that my current email address still uses some of those numbers!

Mark recognised that the ability to judge risk effectively was the essence of his pre-morbid success as an underwriter, and that his ability to do this depended upon picking up on and remembering pieces of information about locations such as earthquake zones and oil spills, as well as high- and low-risk companies. To compensate for his memory difficulties in relation to this issue, he developed a database of information about insurance risks (i.e. details of major losses/disasters compiled from the Lloyds list of such losses). This was in order to keep up to date with information to which he could refer when assessing risk associated with new business. Many of these strategies might be used by the non-memory-impaired underwriter, but Mark had previously been successful without needing to refer to them. For this reason he had to go through the process of appreciating the nature of his difficulties, accepting the need for memory aids, implementing strategies and evaluating their value. There was a risk of Mark developing depressive symptoms as his insight increased, so managing the emotional component of his rehabilitation was important, and this was achieved by psychological support though group sessions and occasional individual support (for more on emotion, mood and rehabilitation see Wilson, Gracey, Evans & Bateman, 2009).

Goal 2: To identify whether he can return to his previous employment

Mark's top priority was to return to work. He knew that he needed to demonstrate a broad range of underwriting skills and knowledge in order to be considered for a return to his pre-injury position with his employers. Their policies were strict in the face of worldwide losses that required the need to make good decisions regarding new insurance agreements. He also knew that he needed to maintain relationships with brokers.

Goal 3: To demonstrate competence in negotiation skills as rated by a work colleague

Two senior managers from the firm came to the OZC to establish a plan for Mark's staged return to work by which his progress from each stage would be judged according to his demonstration of key insurance and underwriting skills. Critical to Mark's successful return to work was, we believe, this programme of step-wise increases in the level of work responsibilities. He began by returning to work one day each week and this was increased gradually to four days a week. Initially he shadowed other underwriters, who would ask him for his views on business offered to them by brokers. Mark needed to demonstrate appropriate awareness of the issues raised in making agreements, and a short-term goal for reaching this stage was achieved in the time set.

The second stage involved Mark completing limited underwriting tasks, such as mid-term adjustments, and this represented a further short-term goal. He achieved this goal too. Achieving these goals required Mark to continue to develop systems for managing his work.

Next he undertook 'minimal risk' business such as insurance renewals. This goal was not achieved in the time set due to lack of opportunity (because of lack of business) and not, according to Mark's manager, because of difficulties in showing technical knowledge needed for being in an underwriting role. The manager felt that another two weeks were needed to enable him to establish, with Mark, the criteria for the fourth stage of his return to work. He further noted that he wished to broaden the criteria established for the third stage of Mark's work re-entry to include issues relating to marketing products as this was likely to increase business opportunities. He further noted that these were skills that Mark was particularly good at prior to his injury. The manager agreed to meet Mark weekly to review progress. After this, Mark was able to make underwriting decisions as long as they were checked by his manager.

Finally, Mark was given full underwriting authority. The positive reports received from his manager at work suggested that Mark coped with the level of work undertaken, showing insight into the value of using strategies to help cope with difficulties as they arose. Furthermore, as the level of work increased, Mark continued to be vigilant to the possibility of cognitive difficulties impacting on his work and implemented strategies as necessary. For the last three months of the programme Mark attended work five days a week. The staged approach to return to work was necessary for a variety of reasons. It allowed his manager to develop confidence in Mark's judgement in a high-risk business. It enabled Mark to develop his confidence. It also allowed time for Mark to learn to apply the strategies he had developed to compensate for memory problems.

Seven months after the start of his rehabilitation programme, i.e 16 months after his accident, Mark was reinstated on the company payroll, and 14 years later he remains employed. He continues to use the strategies he learned, which he reports are absolutely necessary to his success at work. By being in work he contributes to the cost of his rehabilitation through the tax he pays on his salary and through the tax his company pays as a result of Mark's success in his work. By being in work, welfare costs are also saved. Not all patients undertaking rehabilitation are in a position to make such clinical or financial gains. While it might seem unethical to judge the value of rehabilitation by its cost-effectiveness, cases such as Mark's illustrate that rehabilitation can be both clinically effective *and* cost-effective.

Goal 4: To manage his financial affairs independently

Mark adopted a financial management system that has enabled him to stay in credit in his bank account. He worked out each month how much income went into his bank account, how much left his account for standing orders and direct debits, and then he allocated what was left to spend on a daily or weekly basis. He was able to keep within this limit. He discussed with the occupational therapist how he would manage unexpected events and how he would proceed once his debts had been cleared, although he was reluctant to pursue a system where he could account for *every* penny he spent. For the whole of the programme and for the following year during his follow-up reviews, Mark remained in credit.

Goal 5: To develop a range of leisure interests that benefit his memory functioning

Mark identified a list of activities that he wished to pursue, including racing his mountain bike, achieving his yachtsman's qualifications and learning Italian. He was encouraged to explore what problems he may encounter in pursuing these activities, and to prioritise which, and when, to pursue. Mark continued to pursue his interest in mountain biking, and took responsibility for organising events for his local club. He also registered himself and participated in a yachting course. He enrolled on an Italian course, which he started in November 1998. He monitored how well he was able to balance the demands of coursework while returning to work. During the months following his discharge, Mark discontinued his Italian classes, which he had undertaken for interest and for the demand it would have on his memory. He stopped the classes because of lack of time once he was back at work full time. Despite this, Mark managed to maintain a very active physical regime of working out, running and cycling. He also started other activities, such as cycle orienteering, which made demands on his planning and memory skills.

In short, Mark had achieved all his goals and managed to return to a demanding job. More importantly, he has remained employed ever since.

I adjusted to life at the Oliver Zangwill Centre; I stayed at a guesthouse in Ely Sunday to Thursday night returning home on Friday night. I joined a gym in Ely, attended talks and film showings at the Maltings and generally my life revolved around Ely. I would hasten to say that being single suited this lifestyle as, if I'd had to balance my rehabilitation with family life, it would've put undue pressure on me at a time when I was able to focus totally on my cognitive work.

I was extremely fortunate in that a Lloyds broker (with whom I used to conduct a lot of business pre-crash) was able to come up to the Oliver Zangwill Centre a couple of times to broke 'mock business' to me in a replication of how we transact business in the Lloyds market as, although everyone is aware of insurance, the way that business is transacted on a face-to-face basis in Lloyds is quite unique. I thought that it was very important that the staff at the centre took the steps to re-enact my work trading environment and then asked the broker whether he thought that my responses were on par with 1) the decisions that I might have made before or 2) in line with what other underwriters might make?

Life at the centre was very structured; you always knew what you were meant to be doing and where you were meant to be doing it. Another important aspect of the centre was being with other clients and, even though they might have different injuries or disabilities or be at different stages of their time at the centre, there was always a strong bond between us all. There were several clients at the centre during my time there and the fact that some of them were staying in the same guest house or walked the same way to the centre as you gave you a good feeling of camaraderie with them or, in my instance, someone to chat to in the evenings or play squash with. One of my highlights at the centre was organising a trip for the other clients to the horse-racing museum at Newmarket.

Jonathan Evans and others at the centre liaised with my company about a gradual return to employment back into my previous role and I was taken off permanent health insurance and re-employed as an underwriter on 13 January 1999 (16 months after my accident).

As for my life now, I'm a Lloyds underwriter writing worldwide property business in the Lloyds Building in Lime Street. I'm married with two daughters and although I no longer coach each week, the club that I helped set up seven years ago (Go-Ride Bexley) still attracts 20 to 25 young riders each week and many of them have now joined the Woolwich Cycling Club (that I chair) and are regularly racing in and around London and the South East.

In 1998 I went back to Sion in Switzerland, in the year after the crash, with my mother and sister to meet and thank the surgeons (Professor Ravisson was one I seem to remember) and the other staff who had saved my life the year before.

The surgeons knew that I was coming but some of the medical staff didn't and were slightly taken aback to see me walking and talking as they told me later that 'for a few weeks we thought that you were going to die, Mark' – that really gave me some insight as to how grave my condition had been in 1997.

I rode in the Alps again in 2000 and then completed the entire 'ill-fated' Tour de Mont Blanc in 2001. I was fortunate to be able to ride with one of the guys that I was riding with on my crash day in 1997; he was in fact the guy who climbed down the mountain to save me and had called in the mountain rescue and had (so he says) sang to me to get some sort of response until the helicopter arrived! Simon and I have remained good friends and are still in contact to this day.

I think that the realisation of the full extent of my injuries/disabilities whilst in a session with Jonathan Evans at the centre was a pivotal point of my recovery; as only when I was fully aware of exactly what I could and couldn't do was I able to work on the strategies explained by Huw Williams and the rest of the team to help compensate in the areas that I was lacking.

The cycle coaching club that I set up several years ago is going from strength to strength. We now have anything up to 30 children aged between 7 and 16 every Saturday. The older ones have now joined the Woolwich Cycling Club (of which I'm Chairman) and 12 of us rode a 100-km reliability trial in Kent recently! One of the older boys absolutely 'wiped the floor' with me whilst riding yesterday as I was really struggling up the last few hills! To give you some idea of how tough this was my GPS device showed that I burnt 4,750 calories over 65 miles with 750 metres of climbing – wow!

Jolanta Ossetin sadly died in 2009. I spoke at her memorial service on 18 September 2009. I said I was very pleased to speak about someone who was a key driver in my recovery. I mentioned how tough she was on me at the Devonshire and also how she pushed for me to attend the OZ Centre to complete my recovery. I am really glad she did.

Chapter 15

Vicky's story

'Lifting the stone eggs from my heart'

Fiona Ashworth and Vicky Prouten

Vicky was a young woman enjoying the freedom of living her life independently and having fun with her friends. She was a lovely person and loved her family deeply, always putting them first. She also took good care of herself, and could be described as being a perfectionist in all aspects of her life. However, things changed very suddenly for this determined young woman when she was involved in a car accident after a night out with friends.

Introduction

Vicky was a 28-year-old woman living with her boyfriend in Jersey. A high-spirited woman, she was close to her family and enjoyed spending time with family and friends. She was a very hard worker and liked to get things right. She liked keeping fit and had plans to study childcare at a local college.

Before the car crash I'd had a good job in finance, booking business travel. Since I left school, I'd had an absolute ball whilst sharing a flat with a friend, and I'd even had two jobs at the same time – one full-time and the second one an evening job to support my lifestyle and make ends meet.

In 2004, I'd moved back home with my mum to save money so I could take time out to go travelling. In 2005, I went travelling by myself and, after two trips away, I was on such a high and I finally found some focus for my future and realised that on my return home I wanted to do my A-levels at a local college to enable me to go on to university to become a nurse.

I enrolled to do my A-levels in the May, and in September of 2005 I was starting my studies. It really was happy days, I felt empowered and excited for the future. Not to forget the fun side of that year, spending a lot of time with my friends enjoying nights out socialising. From the short statement above I hope I managed to get across the type of person I was back then. I was fiercely independent, determined (some might say stubborn), strong-willed and focused. Little did I know that my happy days and ultimately my whole life were going to change forever.

Background of injury

In October 2005 I was a passenger involved in a horrific car crash. I sustained many injuries, the worst being a serious brain injury. The aftermath of that night in October was and still is to this day very difficult to cope with. First came my release from hospital two months after the crash itself. I got home being so pleased to be out of hospital that I just assumed life would return to normal. Luckily, my mum was able to take time off work to be at home with me for the first few weeks to check that I was OK and coping. I'd not long come out of post-traumatic amnesia, which had lasted six weeks, and I had no insight into the reality of what had happened to me. I was told that this was a classic repercussion of brain injury.

Having no insight into my situation threw up many problems for me. I was able to accept that I'd need to drop out of my A-levels, but I couldn't fathom why I didn't feel right in my head, I felt different to how I felt before. I didn't know who I was, not literally, but I didn't know how I fitted into the world anymore.

When it came to things I'd done before, things that were securely saved in my long-term memory like catching the bus to go into town, I was able to still be independent, thankfully. As the months went on I was desperately searching for something familiar, something that reminded me of who I was before. I found it in the form of my old job booking business travel, and in as little as ten months after my brain injury I was back at work. It was what I wished for in the sense of being familiar, however instead of it reminding me of who I used to be, therefore who I was now, all it did was highlight what I'd lost since my brain injury.

As time was going on I was gaining insight into what had happened to me and, more seriously, I was beginning to become painfully aware of all of the difficulties I was having because of the damage to my brain. As a self-confessed perfectionist, it was horrendous, especially as pre-brain injury me was able to float through life with ease and work to the highest standard and not make mistakes. Post-brain injury me had slowed speed of information processing and I had problems with my attention, short-term memory, planning, problem solving, organisation and communicating with people. I had problems with every skill I needed to do my job. I suffered terribly with fatigue and in turn that made my difficulties worse, it was soul destroying.

Vicky was 21 years old when she was a restrained passenger involved in a road traffic accident on 7 October 2005. At the scene of the accident, her Glasgow Coma Scale (GCS) was recorded as 3/15, but had risen to 11/15 on admittance to the hospital's emergency department. Over the next half hour her GCS fell to 9 and she was intubated and ventilated. Vicky also suffered a number of orthopaedic injuries. A CT scan carried out shortly after she arrived at the hospital noted cerebral oedema with petechial haemorrhages. A further CT scan 24 hours later indicated diffuse axonal injury but no other focal abnormalities. Post-traumatic amnesia was estimated to be for some weeks.

Prior to the accident, Vicky had been living independently in her own flat in Jersey but had only just moved back home to live with her divorced mother and her younger brother who has cerebral palsy. Vicky's family were supportive and she was close to them, especially her mother and grandmother.

Vicky not only struggled with her job after her injury, she also struggled outside work with managing her mood, which was often low. As part of a legal case regarding the accident, Vicky saw a specialist medical consultant on the mainland who referred her to the Oliver Zangwill Centre (OZC) for further assessment and possible rehabilitation.

By the time the opportunity came up to go to the Oliver Zangwill Centre for reha-bilitation I was absolutely fully aware of the differences between pre-brain injury me and post-brain injury me and the comparison was too painful to bear and it was starting to have a negative effect on me. I was massively anxious all of the time, which caused me to develop a negative relationship with food, which made me binge eat, I smoked more and drank more alcohol too. I felt like I was drowning, I couldn't do it anymore, but no way would I admit that to myself, so what do I do? I push myself harder at work and pretend it's not happening.

Assessment

Vicky was assessed at the OZC almost two years after her accident. She saw a team of psychologists, occupational therapists and speech and language therapists in order to obtain a holistic and comprehensive view of her strengths and challenges post-injury.

Cognitive assessment

Neuropsychological assessment highlighted difficulties in the domains of speed of processing, attention and executive functioning. In partic-ular, Vicky had difficulties with goal management, shifting attention and self-monitoring, and poor prospective memory.

Mood assessment

From a psychological perspective, Vicky was struggling with very low self-esteem, symptoms of depression and anxiety and binge eating in response to her low self-esteem. She described herself as a 'ruminator', often focusing on negative thoughts and perceptions and finding it hard to shift her attention away from them, and this rumination often led her to feel anxious.

Social communication assessment

Vicky showed communication difficulties including low assertiveness and miscommunications in conversations such as 'getting the wrong end of the stick'.

Functional assessment

Vicky was struggling to cope at work, was often forgetful and easily distracted and struggled to solve problems. This often led to increased anxiety and stress, exacerbating both cognitive and psychological difficulties. Socially, Vicky had become increasingly isolated from friends, as she did not feel confident interacting with them. Often she was critical of herself, ruminating about what might happen if she said the wrong thing or what people might think of her since the brain injury. She had managed to continue her relationship with her boyfriend, but at times found it difficult to communicate openly about how she was feeling, as she was often confused about her emotions.

Physical considerations

Physical problems were also noted, including heightened fatigue and amenorrhea, which may have been linked to endocrinology changes as a direct result of the brain injury.

A diagrammatic formulation of Vicky's interacting difficulties is highlighted in Figure 15.1. It was evident to the team that Vicky could benefit from holistic neuropsychological rehabilitation and she was therefore recommended for the programme.

Rehabilitation

Vicky returned just weeks after her assessment in late 2007 to start the programme. Given that Vicky was moving to Cambridgeshire from

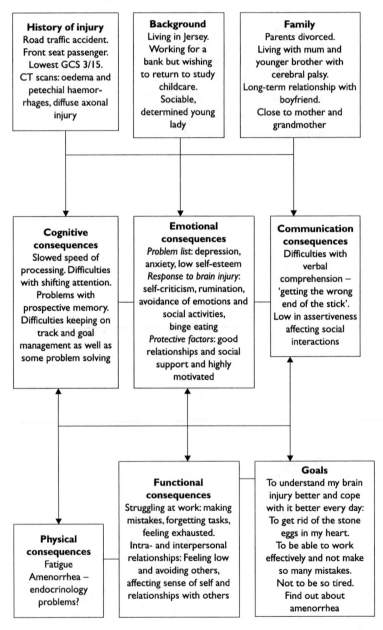

Figure 15.1 Vicky's formulation.

Jersey for the six months of the programme, the team was mindful of ensuring she had the support she needed. In fact, her boyfriend Steve decided he would move to Cambridgeshire with her for the six months. With the support of our administration team, Vicky and her boyfriend found a flat close to the OZC and comfortable for the two of them. Progress, outcome and family meetings were arranged in advance in order that the family could find the most suitable dates to come to Cambridgeshire and make the best of the time at the centre. In order to be flexible, the outcome meeting was arranged in Jersey after the programme had finished so that the team could meet with Vicky's wider support system including her employer. With Vicky's permission, regular contact was made via telephone with her employer and family throughout the programme.

Vicky was now ready to start the programme. Interestingly, hers was the first ever completely female cohort. Vicky attended with four other women, all of whom had some commonalities with regard to the consequences of their injuries including low assertiveness and low self-esteem. This meant that the programme could be tailored to gender-specific issues.

It was just over two years since the car crash when I started rehabilitation. It was a breath of fresh air for me, it was my only glimmer of hope that I desperately needed to cling on to. Rehabilitation was hard, but for me real life back home was ten times harder so I embraced every moment of rehabilitation. The first few weeks of it made me feel very vulnerable, the process felt mentally and emotionally invasive, but as time went on all the pieces of the jigsaw seemed to fit and it all began to make sense. I felt that the harder I worked during rehabilitation then the more my brain would heal, and if I was lucky I might just catch a glimpse of that independent young lady that I used to be. I found out so much about myself and for that I feel blessed. It was wonderful to have the support of the other clients on the course as well as the support and experiences of previous clients.

Vicky and her therapy team set the following goals.

Goal 1: Vicky will develop an understanding of the cognitive, communication, emotional and functional consequences of her brain injury

Vicky was particularly interested in understanding more about endocrinology functioning. Second, she wanted to develop strategies to manage her challenges. She wanted to become more aware of her emotions, improve her self-esteem, become more assertive, manage her fatigue and manage her goals and her attention better.

Understanding more about her endocrinology (particularly with regards to her amenorrhea)

Vicky had reported her concerns that she had not had her period since her injury. In particular, she was concerned about not being able to have children in the future. Initially, she learned more about endocrine function through group and one-to-one sessions and how brain injury may impact on this. Vicky was then referred to a local neurologist who determined that she needed further assessment at the endocrine clinic to find out if there were problems related to the brain injury. The assessment found no problems with regard to endocrine functioning linked to fertility, but it did indicate heightened cortisol levels (a stress response hormone) and she was advised to continue psychological work on managing stress.

Vicky attended Understanding Brain Injury (UBI) groups, including those for Mood, Cognition, Communication and Support, and individual sessions with the team. These sessions helped her to understand the consequences of her injury and develop ways to manage these so that she could take part in her life in a way that was less effortful and left her feeling more contented. Each section below outlines the rehabilitation programme goals and the progress that Vicky made in each area.

Goal 2: Vicky will develop a greater awareness of her emotions

In the initial psychotherapy sessions, Vicky developed an understanding of her psychological difficulties. Her psychologist helped her to increase her understanding of what she was experiencing emotionally in different situations and to communicate these feelings. We used a basic cognitive behavioural approach that taught Vicky to monitor her thoughts, feelings and behaviours in given situations and reflect on these in psychotherapy sessions. It became apparent that Vicky was able to label her feelings, but she had a tendency to try to avoid expressing them, particularly when they were difficult. She reflected that although it initially felt more effortful to focus on and report her feelings, it was a cathartic process and she felt that it worked better than trying to avoid and 'box' them.

Goal 3: Vicky will improve her self-esteem through learning to be more compassionate to herself

Vicky developed a key understanding of her low self-esteem. An historical perspective indicated that Vicky had struggled with low self-esteem prior to her accident and this had been exacerbated by the injuries. At the centre of her difficulties was a belief that 'I am not worthwhile' with highly self-critical thoughts cascading from this about herself and her abilities, which also contributed to high levels of anxiety and symptoms of depression. Vicky aptly described her psychological state as 'having stone eggs in my heart'.

Initially, she and her psychologist worked to improve her self-esteem and reduce symptoms of anxiety and depression through a cognitive behavioural framework. However, therapy reached a 'sticking point' when she reflected that she did not consider she was improving as although she *believed* she was a 'worthwhile person', she did not *feel* it. Therefore, a compassion focused re-formulation was developed with Vicky through Compassion Focused Therapy (CFT; Gilbert, 2005, 2010a, 2010b), including using Compassionate Mind Training (CMT) adapted in the context of acquired brain injury. Vicky found the use of compassionate imagery particularly useful, developing an image of a 'compassionate ideal' or 'perfect nurturer' (Lee, 2005). Details of this compassion-focused intervention can be found in a recent publication (Ashworth, Gracey & Gilbert, 2011).

Goal 4: Vicky will improve her social confidence and assertiveness through assertiveness training

Vicky began to make sense of her lack of self-confidence in being assertive with others in the context of her psychological formulation and interacting consequences of her brain injury. In the Communication Group, she gained knowledge as to how to be assertive and she wished to incorporate this into specific interactions with others. The speech and language therapist collaboratively developed a number of prospective situations that offered Vicky the opportunity to test out her new assertiveness skills and see if she could stimulate change in others by changing her communication style.

Using a behavioural experiment approach (Bennett-Levy *et al.*, 2004), Vicky talked through each scenario, made predictions about her performance and the outcome, reflected afterwards on how she had communicated and suggested any changes for further situations. Through this process, she began to appraise the situations more accurately (with less of a negative bias) and noted an increase in confidence in assertively stating what she wanted or how she felt in a given situation. Amongst her achievements, Vicky successfully chaired a busy community meeting at the OZC, as well as chairing her outcome meeting with staff and work colleagues. Vicky reflected that in addition to becoming more assertive, she found the planning ahead in these situations to be very useful.

Goal 5: Vicky will develop strategies to manage her fatigue more effectively

As part of the intensive phase, Vicky received education in both group and individual settings on fatigue as a consequence of brain injury and its impact on everyday life. Vicky and her occupational therapist developed a fatigue formulation (Malley & Cooper, 2006) through regular monitoring of patterns of fatigue, noting what stimulated them, and noting subsequent helpful and unhelpful responses to weariness. As part of this process, Vicky was provided with a useful leaflet called 'Managing Fatigue after Brain Injury' (Cooper & Malley, 2008). She and her therapist developed fatigue management strategies, including pacing and planning, to help her manage her fatigue on a daily basis. Although Vicky demonstrated an ability to implement these strategies, her coping style of pushing herself needed to be closely monitored in order to prevent this from leading to excessive fatigue. Alongside this, Vicky was referred to a Sleep Clinic for assessment of sleep difficulties likely impacting on fatigue. As a result, a trial of Modafinil was recommended to help Vicky feel more awake during the day.

Goal 6: Vicky will develop compensatory strategies to enable her to manage the cognitive consequences of her injury

Attention and goal management

Vicky had reported that she was easily distracted at work by both internal (e.g. self-critical thoughts) and external (e.g. people talking whilst she is working) distracters that also affected her ability to hold things in mind (working memory), leading to memory failures. Vicky learned a number of different compensatory strategies to help her overcome these difficulties, particularly at work. Monitoring highlighted that Vicky particularly struggled to shift her attention from emotional thoughts, so she was introduced to attention training techniques (ATT; Wells, 2008). This became a strategy to help her to shift from an internal focus (e.g. self-critical thoughts) to an external focus and back to the task at hand. The ATT were seen as a way of helping Vicky to view thoughts and feelings and choosing not to respond to them. At the end of the programme, she had more control of her attention and felt that her ability to switch her attention was much more 'snappy'. She developed a cue card to remind her to practise her ATT, which also acted as a reminder of how to switch her attention.

Vicky also worked on developing tools to hold important things in mind (e.g. 'I must do that paperwork in a minute' or 'I must buy some coffee once I have been down the cereal aisle'). She adapted the internal strategy of using a mental blackboard by imagining it as a felt-board on which she stuck pictures of the things she needed to remember. She found this helpful in remembering things in the moment.

Developing a memory and planning system

Vicky's cognitive and occupational therapists worked with her to develop an external memory and planning system to improve daily organisation in order that she could successfully achieve the tasks she set out to achieve each day. Evidence supports the effectiveness of such systems in reducing memory and planning failures in everyday life such as those Vicky was experiencing (Wilson, Emslie, Quirk & Evans, 2001). Her system took the form of a smartphone, which she learned to use effectively to plan and organise her week. She used this to remind herself to practise her rehabilitation strategies by setting herself alerts to the required times. Vicky also learned to use the calendar, to-do list and notes functions on her phone. She planned to synchronise her phone with her computer when she returned to Jersey at the end of the programme.

Goal 7: Vicky will use compensatory strategies to be more effective at work as well as develop a clear vocation action plan

One of Vicky's key reasons for attending rehabilitation was her desire to become more effective in her current work role and to develop a clear vocational action plan for the forthcoming year. The first part of the programme focused on helping her recognise the factors impacting on her ability to complete tasks at work efficiently and effectively. She then worked with different members of the team, especially her occupational therapist, to develop strategies to achieve her roles and responsibilities more fully.

Her employer was 'on board' with the rehabilitation programme and, at the first meeting with her managers, the interacting cognitive, physical and emotional difficulties that had impacted on Vicky and her performance at work were discussed. She then returned to work two days per week. Feedback from Vicky, her line manager, and her treating team offered the opportunity to evaluate her work skills. As a result of this, adaptations were made, including relocating her desk area (so fewer distractions were present) and re-organising her work environment. Continuous positive and constructive feedback provided the opportunity for ongoing 'tweaks' that needed to be made so that Vicky could fulfil her work roles. In the short term, she decided that she wished to continue to work at her current place of employment in order to save enough money to go travelling. Longer term, Vicky reflected that she might wish to take on a vocation, possibly in basic engineering or supporting people with disabilities. However, she was not clear on this yet and decided to consider these options during the review period at the OZC.

Outcome

Vicky made excellent progress during rehabilitation. Her mood improved significantly with increases in her self-esteem to within the normal range as well as a decrease in symptoms of anxiety and depression. She was observed to be considerably more assertive in observable situations and rated herself as more confident in being assertive with others. She found the compensatory cognitive strategies that worked for her, and in particular the smartphone became 'like another limb'. Vicky continued to progress well in her job and reported much higher job satisfaction and job performance after the programme in comparison to before. Vicky continued to face a number of challenges after the programme, but felt that her strategies and particularly her 'star angel' (her compassionate other) helped her through difficult times. Just over two years after finishing at the OZC, Vicky realised her dream and went abroad travelling again. We were really pleased to receive a postcard from her stating how happy she was to have finally met her final goal!

In the four years since rehabilitation I have been re-building my life. In the months immediately after I was on a high, as life all of a sudden was very different to the way it was before rehab. The strategies I'd learnt to help me with my difficulties were working and life in general was easier. A lot of it was to do with the fact rehabilitation had given me the insight into what had happened to my brain because of the damage, and I was finally able to understand it.

My return to work was equally positive, but as time went on I was coming down from the high I felt after rehabilitation. Suddenly things weren't as positive as they seemed at first. As much as I tried I just couldn't avoid the fact that every day in that job I was still comparing my abilities to how they were pre-brain injury and post-brain injury. To add to that, we were short-staffed at work and we were insanely busy. As you can imagine, my anxiety sky-rocketed, which made my difficulties worse and this lasted at least a year or so. In order to cope, I did my usual and I smoked, drank more and my binge eating was getting worse, yet I was losing weight and my health really started to suffer. I was signed off by my GP for a few months to enable me to recover. After much heartache, in the end I left that job and went travelling with a very dear friend of mine. We had the time of our lives and I'll say to this day that that trip saved me. At present, I have a little job in retail which tides me over whilst I'm training in childcare studies at college. I quit smoking two years ago and I no longer drink much alcohol. Can you see my halo, it might slip off if I'm not careful!! My emotional relationship with food is much better, now I see food as nutrition for my body, and not an emotional plug to force all those negative emotions back into those stone eggs which used to weigh down my heart. At the moment I'm trying to come to terms with the fact that re-building my life will be a constant work in progress, I'll not wake up one morning and it'll all be over. I'll never be who I was before the car crash but at least I've stopped looking for her now. I'm beginning to look forward to a different kind of future.

Chapter 16

Robert's story
Understanding is key to invisible injuries

Jill Winegardner and Robert Runcie

Robert was a high-flying workaholic when a cerebellar stroke left him . . . intelligent, articulate, personable. Underneath the normal exterior lurked massive fatigue, pain and hyperacusis (hypersensitivity to sounds) that Robert was at a loss to understand himself, much less explain to friends and family. His eventual solution? Studying his brain and creating a credit-card sized image of his brain to share!

Introduction

I was aged 52, settled with a family and established in a senior position at work. I worked hard and travelled widely, with recent trips to China and Australia. I enjoyed holidays with a difference (environmental and cultural), having been recently to Costa Rica. I was fit and healthy with no past history of sickness.

Background of injury

On 22 April 2010, I was on the train returning from work in London and looking forward to dinner with my wife, Elisabeth. Having ignored an unusually blinding headache the evening before and feeling slightly unwell in the taxi, ten minutes into the journey I became violently ill, vomiting, had difficulty standing, felt dizzy, had hot and cold sweats and was unsteady on my feet. I thought I had food poisoning. On arrival at my destination I was unable to stand unaided, could not cope with the movement of people, struggled to get off the train and could not understand why I found it hard to walk. A train guard helped me across the station to a seat in the ticket hall. My mind was clear but my body had stopped responding.

Luckily an old acquaintance found me and waited until his wife appeared to pick him up. I lurched uncontrollably to the left and within a few small steps, could progress no further. I borrowed my friend's phone to ring my wife, having remembered our number, whilst they drove me to the local 'walk in' centre. I was wheel-chaired in, head spinning, excruciating headaches, double vision, vomiting and slumped to the left with extremely high blood pressure. My wife and son appeared and I knew I was going to be all right (no logic to this, just my belief).

I was admitted to hospital where I spent the next eight days. After three days of tests the neurologists confirmed I'd had a cerebellar stroke – an acquired brain injury. For the first few days I was unable to get out of bed or stand. Luckily my vision returned, and I could hear and speak clearly. I still had excruciating head-aches. With the support of the physiotherapists I managed to move very slowly on a Zimmer frame, progressing quickly to using a walking stick.

After being taught how to manage stairs, I was discharged. At this stage I was not fit to look after myself and relied totally on the support of my wife. I thought that the only barrier to resuming my life as I knew it was the physical impairments of the stroke (how wrong I was on this assumption).

In the first few weeks, intense physiotherapy and lots of exercising, supervised by my wife at home every day, produced outstanding results on getting me back on my feet. However, these benefits had to be offset by the difficulties I now had struggling with noise and visual distraction. I still had intense head pain, I could not watch television, listen to the radio or read a book, and my left side was weaker than my right. I had co-ordination and balance problems, and the left side of my head was numb. Even with a cane, walking was slow, nowhere near straight and standing still very difficult – impossible with my eyes closed. Coming home I real-ised that my brain attack had been much more severe than I realised. I was totally exhausted, sleeping at least 12 hours a night but still waking up fatigued.

As the months passed by, head pains reduced. I found reading personal experi-ences of other stroke survivors was so valuable in comprehending my own situa-tion. So much to learn! I had lots of 'notions'. Often I would wake up and feel normal. I struggled to accept that I was recovering from a serious illness. It felt at times like it had happened to someone else, not me. I am still the same person with the same intellect and humour – just slower.

I am lucky to have the love and 100% support of my wife. My hospital consultant, GP and local support stroke coordinators, the physiotherapy and ongoing exercises to improve my balance and coordination have given me an outstanding physical recovery to date. Less clear and understood are the unseen impacts on my brain. Nine months after my stroke I believed I would soon return to work, but I was not physically or mentally fit enough.

The physiotherapy and clinical support for my recovery was (I believed at the time) very good. What I didn't realise was that the psychological impact of my brain attack was much, much bigger than I could recognise or even comprehend. I now know that I needed the same degree of support I'd had from my doctors and physiotherapists to help me sort out my mental condition.

My cerebellar stroke led to problems with balance, some unilateral weakness and difficulties with attention and concentration. Additionally, I had become highly sensitised to background noise and found it difficult to cope in situations where there were a couple of people and where more than one person may be talking at once. Significant – and at times overwhelming – fatigue has also been a problem for me. Whilst I had been able to regain the ability to walk and climb stairs, these functions now required more conscious effort on my part. This partly explained why I found it difficult to deal with distractions – e.g. when walking it was difficult to attend to conversations, or with people approaching on the pavement when so much of my attention was needed to maintain my ability to continue walking safely. This need to consciously direct my attention towards safe walking ability in turn contributed to my extreme tiredness.

Fatigue that is caused by any type of brain injury – such as my stroke – is regarded as being beyond the experience of those who have never experienced such an injury. It is totally overwhelming and is a very real problem that needs to be managed carefully (and still is nearly three years on). It requires me to plan my day, to allow sufficient rest periods after periods of activity (physical or mental). The fatigue also impacts on my balance, and on cognitive functions such as memory and concentration.

It took me many months to accept that my desire to 'get back to normal as quickly as possible' was actually counter-productive. It was particularly evident when I was overdoing things and subsequently becoming too tired to function well afterwards for several days. My brain did relearn how to do things and the best model for this was a short activity with repeatability – a better model to learn from when my brain can perform well and learn – rather than respond to my insistence on keeping going even when I was clearly exhausted and my performance was suffering and undoing the learning.

It is easy to become disheartened by experiences of overdoing things but I did find that my positive attitude was a huge asset as long as it was used to set realistic goals and challenged me little by little rather than a lot! I got very angry, had uncharacteristic outbursts of temper several times a week and found the loss of personal control of everyday things very difficult to manage.

The assessment by an Addenbrooke's Hospital consultant in rehabilitation medicine identified from my MRI scan an extensive infarct in the cerebellum, and a small area of ischaemia in the left posterior medulla, and on diffusion weighted imaging there was another small abnormality in the right cerebellum. I didn't understand what this really meant until I received in-depth personal feedback at the Oliver Zangwill Centre (OZC) in Ely. I was also referred to the Sleep Laboratory at Papworth Hospital where I was given advice about managing my fatigue – the importance of pacing my days and taking quality rest/sleep periods, e.g. 30 minutes in the morning and 30 minutes in the afternoon before 4pm.

I wanted to go back to being how I was and to my original job. I now realise that this was not realistic. To carry out the job as I used to do it would need lots of adaptations. Being a Board Director of a national company I could not contemplate going back to the same company doing a lesser role. Trying to resolve the uncertainty of future employment didn't help with my rehabilitation!

The prolonged and uncertain process of dealing with returning, or not, to my employment created additional mental health problems. My physical and mental health deteriorated significantly with the stress I was under. My wife did not want me suffering another stroke due to my unstable and high blood pressure! She was looking for a clinical psychologist to help with cognitive and psychological help to move me forward. She believed if this was available I would better come to terms with my new self.

I was referred to a Psychological Therapies service in January 2011 by the Community Stroke Coordinators team (NHS Peterborough Community Services). It was reported by the referral team that whilst I had made good physical recovery and appeared to be functioning at a high cognitive level, concern was expressed regarding my high levels of fatigue and difficulties in focusing and retaining attention (in particular in busy environments). I had been receiving further support from the stroke coordinating team and had also been assessed by the OZC.

I was specifically referred to the Psychological Therapies team to assist me in coming to terms with all that has happened to me during the last year. There were concerns regarding my difficulty to express painful emotion, occasionally losing my temper, which is uncharacteristic for me, and it was felt that the lack of emotional acceptance of my losses (including the potential future loss of my job) was causing me to feel periods of depressed mood with bouts of generalised anxiety, particularly when thinking about issues regarding return to work. On several occasions I expressed difficulty with containing my anxiety when having to face thinking about returning to work and this had an adverse effect on my ability to process the psychological components of the impact of my brain injury.

I engaged well in psychological therapy and was highly motivated, responding well to the intervention over a four-month period.

Assessment

Robert came to the OZC for an Admissions Assessment to see if our rehabilitation programme would be a good fit for him. While Robert had complex consequences including fatigue, cognitive difficulties and emotional changes, the focus of this chapter is his quest to understand what had happened to him. The key to success was found in his developing a shared understanding of his injury and its consequences with the team. The concept of shared understanding is one of the core components of holistic rehabilitation. It suggests that a combination of evidence-based models and theories combined with the client's and family's own personal views and experiences is essential for successful rehabilitation (Wilson, Gracey, Evans & Bateman, 2009).

I was really pleased to attend the two-day assessment at the Oliver Zangwill Centre. Whilst I found this to be very challenging, it was also a great reassurance to have the first real clear feedback on the complex neuropsychological consequences of my brain injury. The OZC assessment – even if I didn't get on the programme, the assessment was invaluable to understanding what was going on in my head.

Rehabilitation

The major turning point in my recovery was attending the neuropsychological rehabilitation programme at the Oliver Zangwill Centre. I rang for some advice on preparation prior to attending. Andrew Bateman advised me to get as fit as I could as the programme is very demanding – as I was to find out. My enthusiasm and energy in the first two weeks resulted in an unplanned trip to the cardiac ward at Addenbrooke's with a good result in that they sorted out my medication, resulting in a more stable heart condition.

Robert started the rehabilitation programme with two other clients.

The first six weeks of the programme focused on learning about brain anatomy, function and the psychological consequences of brain injury. Not only did I crave this knowledge and understanding, but I needed it to put into context what had happened to me and what I could do about it. Sharing experiences with other brain injury sufferers meant there were lots of 'light-bulb' moments when we could say 'ah, that explains why I do ...' This was so valuable to my recovery and only really possible because of the unique environment of the programme.

It was in these first few weeks that my distractibility, and in particular that to do with background noise, was diagnosed as hyperacusis. Thanks to Leyla's [Roberts speech and language therapist] recommendation, my wife purchased some noise-cancelling earphones which changed my life, once I had accepted wearing them in everyday situations. They have enabled my tolerance to improve and over the months my reliance on them has reduced.

My confidence grew and my enthusiasm manifested itself in ways I would not have previously imagined – for example my tendency to demonstrate learning through cake making and photographic records. I had never baked prior to my brain injury, but as part of my rehabilitation, to do bilateral tasks, it has proved to be fun and enjoyable – part of the new me.

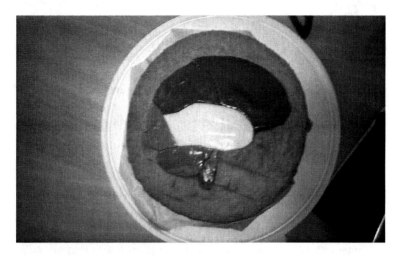

Figure 16.1 Robert's brain cake.

As my understanding and insight to my injury grew I realised that whilst I had started on the journey of acceptance of my brain injury, I was still in denial. This is where the second part of the programme – the integration phase – really came into its own.

The integration phase focused on each of Robert's personal goals in more depth, developing strategies to meet his needs. The team met regularly to assure a shared understanding and coherent and informed planning. Our focus here is on his UBI (Understanding Brain Injury) project.

UBI project

All clients at the OZC are encouraged to create a UBI project to illustrate their journey from injury through rehabilitation. These projects have taken many forms: poetry, music, a garden in the OZC grounds, displays, stories, paintings and more.

My Understanding Brain Injury project had two specific goals:

1   *To understand what had happened to me from an in-depth review of my medical history – in particular the MRI scans.*
2   *To formulate a way of explaining to others my brain injury, as physically I looked very well. Also, as far as others could see, my intellect was unchanged.*

Explaining unseen impacts of brain injuries I found difficult as, in general, people are very wary about discussing mental health.

Part of the problem was me. My natural inclination is to focus on the positives so when someone asked me how I was, I would tell them physically doing really well. My thoughts were also contradictory as I swung from trying to get back to the old me and trying to come to terms with the new me. I could swing mid-sentence and from one conversation to the next giving conflicting views and thoughts. I now know this caused confusion and difficulties for those close to me and those supporting me through the changes at work, hence the need and real value of psychological intervention. Something that has taken until writing this, reviewing what actually happened, and comparing these facts with my recollections which were not always accurate.

I found the time spent reviewing my MRI scans invaluable. To have the detail explained to me so clearly was a revelation. Whilst I understood the impacts of the stroke in my cerebellum affecting balance and co-ordination, I could not or I did not understand what was causing the neuropathic pains I experience daily. And I didn't understand these until Andrew explained that the infarct in my medulla was the cause of Lateral Medullary Syndrome (also called Wallenberg Syndrome). I suppose that whilst knowing the cause didn't mean a cure for it, being able to understand the cause was a tremendous relief. There's something reassuring about knowing the cause of a problem that removes uncertainty, which even without a cure is a weight off my mind.

Robert had daily constant pain on one side of his face that had been labelled as 'neuropathic pain'. This label was not sufficient information for Robert – he asked, 'Why is the pain here?' and, 'What has pain in my face got to do with a stroke?' and, 'Why is it chronic?' Close inspection of the MRI images showed a unilateral wedge-shaped lesion encroaching into the medulla, consistent with the consequences of an occlusion to the posterior inferior cerebellar artery. The lateral medulla is packed with multiple nerve nuclei and tracts, meaning that there is a wide variety of possible constellations of symptoms. For Robert it was sufficient reassurance that readily accessible information on the internet mentioned chronic pain (e.g. Wikipedia entry on Wallenberg Syndrome).

Finding out so much, whilst wonderful in its own right, then needed to be brought into a succinct form for me to use in everyday communication. I created a credit-card sized picture of my brain injury, clearly showing the cerebellar stroke on the left-hand side and on the reverse of the card I summarised the impacts and the consequences as a constant reminder of the new me.

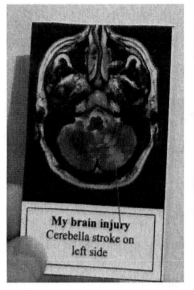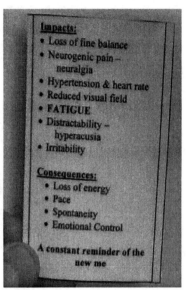

Figure 16.2 Robert's Understanding Brain Injury project.

Not many people can show a picture of the inside of their head.

A friend of mine, who has also suffered a brain injury, commented, 'Most people I know carry a picture of their loved ones in their wallet, you're the only person I've ever met who shows a picture of his brain.'

Like me, this friend finds it extremely frustrating when people say you look really well, just like your old self – makes him feel like sticking a big plaster or bandage on his head.

For me, my brain card has been a turning point in my life as it makes people stop and really think. I use it every time I meet someone new to me.

Outcome

Two and a half years on from my stroke, I am very happy with the new me. I have taken early retirement from my full-time occupation. I do some part-time volun-tary work to stimulate my intellect. My wife and I enjoy our life together and have just completed a major project refurbishing a cottage on the coast, which we found fulfilling. It played a large part in my rehabilitation, allowing us both to focus on doing something together that we enjoyed that wasn't a direct focus on my brain injury. It has improved my stamina, both physically and mentally, enabled me to apply and develop the strategies from OZ – pacing the day, building in rest periods, managing fatigue (still a real problem!), using alarms as a prompt to help attention, 'Stop–Think' (what am I trying to do here? check in on my mental blackboard), simplifying things and being compassionate to myself and others. My reliance on using noise-cancelling earphones has reduced but as the experience of the recent OZC Christmas party showed, I still need to use them in noisy surroundings.

Finally, I recognise the importance of the love and unstinting support by my wife. Not everybody has the energy, intellect and tenacity to search and fight for the professional help she knew I needed.

Chapter 17

Alex's story

Calming the drama and sticking with life

Jill Winegardner and Alexander J. Cowan

We first learned about Alex when his mother phoned the Oliver Zangwill Centre (OZC) to say that her 34-year-old son had impetuously decided to leave his London flat and move back in with his parents in a village in Wiltshire. She was distressed and hoping we might be able to help. Alex came for a visit but became distracted while driving into town, smashed his car, and arrived with a fresh red bleeding knot on his forehead. We were to learn that high drama played a big role in Alex's life, with crises alternating with boredom/depression.

Introduction

Born in London, Alex spent his first four years in the Middle East with his parents. The family returned to a village in Wiltshire where he grew up, the only boy with three older half-sisters and two younger sisters. He attended boarding school in rural Wiltshire from age 11 to 18 and described it as a difficult experience, saying he was bullied and ostracised as a child, likely because he was gay. He described himself as very bright but also very lazy, so he was constantly earning marks that reflected high intellect and poor effort.

After taking a gap year, Alex enrolled in the dental school at the University of London. While a student, he both worked hard and played hard. He said that during these years 'I had it all', doing well academically and having many friends. Things were finally looking up for him.

Background of injury

Alex was in his fifth year of dental school in London when he was struck down by a motorist while walking home and suffered a severe brain injury. He was taken to hospital, where he spent two to three days in the

Intensive Care Unit and another three weeks in the High Dependency Unit. He had a right supraorbital fracture and right frontal petechial haemorrhaging with four weeks of post-traumatic amnesia. Alex then underwent inpatient rehabilitation for five months, was briefly discharged to his parents' home, and then entered a Transitional Living Unit for another seven months. Towards the end of this time, he attempted suicide by overdose and was hospitalised overnight in the main hospital and had a psychiatric evaluation. He was discharged home to his parents soon thereafter and had no further rehabilitation for brain-injury related difficulties except brief physiotherapy and surgery to correct diplopia.

On the occasion of the Diamond Jubilee, while in the midst of rehabilitation, Alex wrote this essay:

The Diamond Jubilee – an alternative standpoint

Nearly 12 years ago I suffered a severe traumatic brain injury (TBI). I was in my fifth and final year of studying dental surgery at Guy's Hospital in London. A TBI is, without any shadow of a doubt, a completely life-changing experience.

'Yes, yes, yes,' you may say. 'We all know, state the obvious, why don't you.' So many people come to one's hospital bedside – family, friends, acquaintances, priests and priestesses, friends of friends, etc., etc. They cry, are angry, shout, scream, cuddle you, kiss you whatever, they are there.

Then comes life. Not the life you remember or indeed enjoyed so much. Not a life of physical pain or even suffering, a life that is made up of simply existing on a day-to-day basis. 'But that's what we all do', you might say. What do I make that mean? To me, that means life does not involve any enjoyment or fun. That is not the life I see of others. For I vicariously live life. Not through all those hospital visitors, no, through the television.

I am convinced therefore that life is not simply a challenge, for it is a challenge for everyone, but a trial set in purgatory. I remember very clearly sitting outside the cable-car in the ski resort my family's been going to since the eighties. There I remember sitting with my mother having a cup of coffee. 'Our poor girls, the poor girls, they've had no life.' What did I make this mean? It was my fault for having a brain injury. It was therefore my fault they'd had no life. I'd had four years of life, therefore I didn't need any more.

I felt I had to do everything I could to make sure my family could appreciate me. Less than a year after a brain injury I was in no physical way able to help anyone, and the only thing I could do was to spend money on them. I chose a banker who'd let me spend my compensation money – almost willy-nilly. One who made no pursing of his lips when I said I wanted to buy my parents a house – all the others had, I never understood why. I do now.

I do not feel the same, I do not think the same, I do not want the same things, I am not the same. And yet the understanding of neurological damage leads to most people in this world (including most doctors) that one comes into contact with regarding one the same way, treating one in the same way, thinking that one thinks the same way and feels the same way.

I know full well that my parents never meant to do anything they did with malice, did everything they did out of love, care and kindness. They would do all they could for their offspring and there should be no primus inter pares (first among equals). What is so difficult for me to swallow is that my family left me alone and isolated. For any illness is an isolating experience, the more serious one's illness or injury, the more serious one's isolation.

My parents had each other, my sisters had each other, my friends (the drunken students they were) had each other. No one ever befriended me. I had no soul-mate, no friend who could even begin to understand, no family member even beginning to wish to know what it was like for me. It is almost like I have been moved off tack to a different plateau. One from which I can merely observe life, never allowed to join in. One whereby I can look at fun, feel people's raucous laughter, even experience the enjoyment of others; see their rosy cheeks, the glint in their eyes, feel the warmness emanating from them. If I am ever in that warmness, if my eyes ever glint, if I laugh or shout (I cannot any longer cry), it is a passing moment. It is something that does not last, or indeed ever will. To accept something follows admitting there is something wrong. Admitting defeat by the 'wrongness' in your life. Something, probably something I've learnt, leads me to believe this is an incorrect course of action.

As I've previously mentioned, no malice was behind any decision taken, and everything was thought of as the best decision AT THE TIME. However, this does not make it the right decision nor what will be the best for the long term. My contact with my family prior to my brain injury was limited, my father provided money as and when, and my mother provided laundry facilities once a month or so. This situation I could manage, brief contact with one's parents. My accident infantilised me, once again I was thrown into the arms of my parents. Very soon, friends from university, friends from school and my siblings were all moving along and getting on with their lives. I was stuck in a limbo.

I had a brain that functioned extraordinarily well but a body that did not. I'd achieved academically but whilst at school, only by the skin of my teeth. Consequently I have grades of academic performance from my adolescence that do not reflect my true abilities. I was admitted to dental school on the basis of my interview. There I achieved more than satisfactorily, in fact even exceeding my own expectations. However, my TBI cut short my academic life and I did not gain my qualification to practise as a dental surgeon.

Not only therefore did I have to face the world with a new (less than fully functioning) body and brain, but I had to find a new and different career from everything (and everybody) I knew. I was almost 23 when my accident occurred. I had 'metaphorically speaking' had my legs taken away. I had a case manager from my local council who wanted to put me in a place planting pots with flowers for rehabilitation.

How would I get myself out of this situation?

In the ten years between his brain injury rehabilitation and the time we met him, Alex really struggled to stay with activities. He attempted both paid and voluntary work, but has not held either for more than a few weeks. He said that he left positions either because he was fired or he got bored, commenting that 'my laziness has been accentuated by my brain injury'. For example, in 2002 he obtained an internship with a consultancy group, but impulsively left after two months and went to San Francisco, staying there only two days. His longest voluntary employment was a position in university administration for a couple of months.

Alex has had better luck with educational ventures. He earned a certificate in a foundation course in psychotherapy and narrowly missed passing a diploma course in journalism in 2007–2008. He described his relative success in education as due to the fact that it was focused, attainable and routine.

In November 2009, Alex ended a long-term relationship and felt hopeless about the future. He attempted suicide by throwing himself under a London tube train. Suicide is unfortunately more common following brain injury (Fleminger *et al.*, 2003; Teasdale and Engberg, 2001). He fractured his back and continues to have back pain to this day. Following the suicide attempt, he underwent voluntary treatment at various residential programmes in the United States and in England, intended to treat alcohol and substance abuse and childhood trauma. He did not feel that these programmes were particularly helpful. In addition, he joined Alcoholics Anonymous (AA) and stopped drinking in October 2004. Finally, he has engaged in substantial private psychotherapy. His psychiatrists have felt that he has suffered depressive episodes in the context of brain-injury related personality change. Alex has felt that, since his brain injury, his ordinary personality features were exaggerated and his emotions were more labile, noting especially increased anger and saying things without thinking them through.

Alex was based in London but travelled extensively in the ten years after his early rehabilitation. He reported that depression was the driving force for much of his travel. In the autumn of 2011, he left his home in

London and moved in with his parents in Wiltshire. He felt desperate for help and decided to look for a rehabilitation programme that addressed brain injury rather than substance abuse or trauma, and decided to give the OZC a try.

Assessment

Alex came to the OZC for a two-day Admissions Assessment to see if we would be a good match for him. On meeting Alex, we found him to be a bright, personable and friendly man. He was generally articulate and well-spoken, though at times he was disinhibited and overly familiar. As a result of his brain injury, he had mild ataxia, tremor, a broad-based gait, a slight facial droop on the right and ataxic yet very intelligible speech. He wore glasses and had on a slightly too small shirt one day, so the buttons tugged. He commented that his weight fluctuates as a result of mood-related impulsive eating and lack of routine exercise. Other physical problems included altered and diminished sense of smell, temperature dysregulation, such that he gets hot very easily, and fatigue.

Alex has really made a remarkable recovery in many ways from a very severe injury. He is completely independent in both personal care and general activities of daily living. He has lived alone and carries out all domestic tasks including shopping, cooking, household chores, laundry, and managing appointments. He manages his own finances but commented that 'I mismanage my finances', acknowledging that he has spent large sums of money perhaps unwisely. He drives independently, though after the accident he had when first visiting us he was advised to take a four-hour driving course, and he has now stopped driving.

Usual activities at the time we met Alex included going to the Apple store for training on his computer, shopping, using the computer for email and research, walking for exercise, socialising with friends and watching a documentary or good series on television in the evening. He had stopped going to the gym.

Alex was in a relationship with a Japanese man from 2007–2009, but he ended the relationship, feeling it was not an equal partnership. He has had casual relationships but would like to have a serious relationship.

Cognitive assessment

Alex told us that his thinking abilities had changed, but it was hard to define in what way. He commented that 'everything feels slightly different'. He noted some trouble tracking conversations, minor forgetfulness, and said that learning and retaining were somewhat harder now. He was aware that he did better with routine. When asked about executive function difficulties, he said that 'planning, organising, problem solving are okay with Citalopram [he takes 40 mg per day], though it's hard to say. I don't know if my forward planning [problem] is due to brain injury or to indecision.' Regarding impulsivity and disinhibition, he said, 'Oh yes, my inappropriate comments! I always was inappropriate but now more so, and then I feel so awful and suicidal after.'

Alex underwent two hours of neuropsychological testing directed at identifying underlying cognitive difficulties resulting from his injury, and targeting areas needing rehabilitation. His academic and vocational history, his articulate use of language and good vocabulary, and test results all indicated that he was an exceptionally bright man. Given the severity of his injury, many of his intellectual capacities were remarkably spared. Nevertheless, cognitive screening revealed difficulties in the domains of attention, memory and executive functioning including emotion-based decision making, inhibition and cognitive flexibility. Although most of his scores fell within the average range, it is important to emphasise that this is considered a significant drop for Alex, whose pre-injury intellectual abilities were estimated to be in the superior range.

Functional assessments

We asked Alex to complete a computer-based task incorporating accessing information from the internet to attend a social event of his choice in Cambridge travelling from Ely. Alex showed good familiarity and understanding of computers, but we observed challenges with executive functions such as planning the task, organising his approach, monitoring for best choices, and spotting and correcting errors. His mental arithmetic was quick and accurate, and he stayed well within budget.

Alex was then accompanied to Ely town centre by a speech and language therapist. He was asked to complete a number of tasks in the town in order to allow observation of his cognitive and communicative abilities in this functional setting. As Alex himself stressed, he is accustomed to carrying out such roles independently in his everyday life. The tasks included purchasing items in the supermarket, finding out about leisure and learning opportunities in Ely, and enquiring about ISA rates in a building society.

Alex carried out the tasks with just a few prompts. Throughout the assessment he was sociable and entertaining, generating conversation on a variety of topics. The chief area of concern was that Alex made comments without thinking them through and then found himself needing to apologise. For example, he commented that one of the items on his list, wafer-thin ham, was 'revolting', and later apologised when he realised it was for the therapist accompanying him. He made comments under his breath about a lady's size and about a point made by a gentleman nearby, but not so they could be heard. Alex referred to a recent altercation over some dog waste, repeating swear words used in the hospital. Staff reported that he had recounted the tale fully in the staff lunch room the previous day, without censoring it himself to take account of the fact that people were eating. While none of these moments gave rise to any problems, it seemed likely that Alex's open style (and at times disinhibition and impulsivity) would lead to difficult situations socially, and Alex himself reported that he 'gets into trouble'. He noted that he blames his brain injury but that it does not usually work as people lack knowledge of such injuries.

Overall, these functional tasks mirrored difficulties with executive functioning that had been identified by Alex and seen on standardised testing.

Mood assessment

In his mood assessment, Alex identified several challenges with mood, relationships and behaviour.

Episodes of depression and suicidality

Alex reflected that he has found it very difficult to adjust to the changes in his life, particularly reflecting that he feels he has a sense of discrepancy regarding where he is currently in life compared to where he feels he would have been if the accident had not happened. Alex was administered the Hospital Anxiety and Depression Scales (HADS), which did not highlight current active symptoms of anxiety or depression.

Negative self-evaluation and negative social comparison

Alex often finds himself comparing himself to others negatively. He reflected that he feels a real sense of social stigma related to the consequences of the TBI, particularly the ataxia. He also reported that he tends to criticise himself repeatedly as a result of this. This negative social comparison has led to Alex developing negative self-beliefs, which have a ruminative quality.

Emotional lability

Alex reported that he is sensitive to significant mood swings, both highs and lows. He reported that he occasionally 'flips out', getting angry with himself or others. He further reported that when he experiences periods of 'high' mood, he can have a sense of grandiosity.

Previous history of alcohol abuse

Impressively, Alex has been able to abstain from alcohol use since 2004, after receiving intensive input for this.

Relationship difficulties

Alex noted that he has difficulties with relationships with his family, although he reported that this dated back to before his TBI. He reflected that he has also struggled to find a lasting intimate relationship since 2009, and is keen to do so.

Our assessment findings were pooled and we created a formulation to help us understand Alex in all of his complexity (see Figure 17.1). We used the formulation to begin to develop his rehabilitation plan.

Rehabilitation – the plan

We agreed that Alex would return to the Oliver Zangwill Centre for the intensive programme. In particular, our focus was to support his overall goal of greater understanding and self-acceptance. In his words, the programme 'offers me the opportunity to really find myself'.

To that end, we anticipated that rehabilitation would address the following aims:

- improve his knowledge and awareness of the consequences of his injury through psycho-education and psychological support;
- provide him with strategies to compensate for his neuropsychological impairments, in particular helping him with specific executive difficulties including identifying and managing his goals as well as support with inhibition;

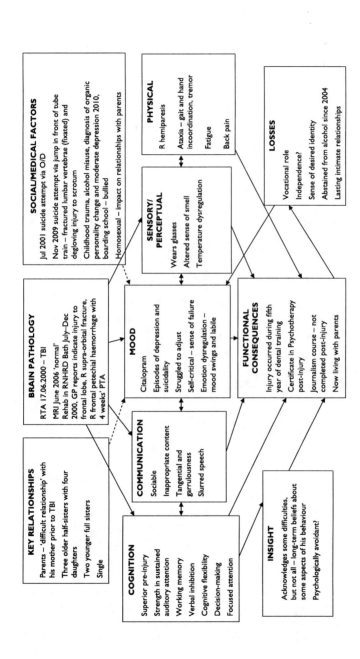

KEY RELATIONSHIPS

Parents – 'difficult relationship' with his mother prior to TBI

Three older half-sisters with four daughters

Two younger full sisters

Single

BRAIN PATHOLOGY

RTA 17.06.2000 – TBI

MRI June 2006 'normal'

Rehab in RNHRD Bath July–Dec 2000, GP reports indicate injury to frontal lobe, R supra-orbital fracture, R frontal petechial haemorrhage with 4 weeks' PTA

SOCIAL/MEDICAL FACTORS

Jul 2001 suicide attempt via jump in front of tube train – fractured lumbar vertebrae (fixated) and degloving injury to scrotum

Childhood trauma, alcohol misuse, diagnosis of organic personality change and moderate depression 2010, boarding school – bullied

Homosexual – impact on relationships with parents

PHYSICAL

R hemiparesis

Ataxia – gait and hand incoordination, tremor

Fatigue

Back pain

SENSORY/ PERCEPTUAL

Wears glasses

Altered sense of smell

Temperature dysregulation

MOOD

Citalopram

Episodes of depression and suicidality

Struggled to adjust

Self-critical – sense of failure

Emotion dysregulation – mood swings and labile

COGNITION

Superior pre-injury

Strength in sustained auditory attention

Working memory

Verbal inhibition

Cognitive flexibility

Decision-making

Focused attention

COMMUNICATION

Sociable

Inappropriate content

Tangential and garrulousness

Slurred speech

FUNCTIONAL CONSEQUENCES

Injury occurred during fifth year of dental training

Certificate in Psychotherapy post-injury

Journalism course – not completed post-injury

Now living with parents

LOSSES

Vocational role

Independence?

Sense of desired identity

Abstained from alcohol since 2004

Lasting intimate relationships

INSIGHT

Acknowledges some difficulties, but not all – long-term beliefs about some aspects of his behaviour

Psychologically avoidant?

Figure 17.1 Alex's formulation.

- address challenges with disinhibition and impulsivity that impede social participation, so that he has the choice to express his personality but also the knowledge and ability to inhibit as appropriate;
- provide psychological support throughout the rehabilitation process, particularly in light of his history of emotional lability and suicide attempts;
- support him in identifying and defining meaningful structured activities of interest and help him find ways to engage in these activities in a sustained and successful manner;
- support his goal of developing and establishing meaningful personal relationships by providing him with increased awareness and understanding of the ways that his brain-injury related difficulties impact on others and by giving him the tools needed to make informed and intentional choices in his interactions with others.

Rehabilitation – the best-laid plans . . .

The plan was that Alex would join a cohort of four men in the Intensive Programme. Unfortunately, our plans went awry. In spite of our best efforts, this particular group did not gel and in fact two group members dropped out of the programme part-way through. From Alex's perspective, he was hoping to meet bright, like-minded people from a similar background to his with similar educational and cultural experiences. Some of the other participants in the group did not engage in the rehabilitation process and were not particularly friendly or sociable. This was highly distressing to Alex, who responded at times with impulsive and angry criticisms of other group members or comments that could be seen as disdainful of them. The cohort eventually disbanded, leaving Alex feeling very disaffected from his rehabilitation and angry with us for not delivering the promised group experience.

We then had a serious re-think about Alex's programme. We went back to the basics of setting goals, and by now we could refine Alex's chief goals along with him, resulting in the following new programme goals:

- find a successful way forward with acceptance of myself . . . meandering through the delta;
- social integration;
- confronting the fear [that if he starts feeling positive, things will surely fall apart].

Our next obstacle was recognising that Alex's goal of social integration was impossible to tackle without the basics being in place: 'Somewhere to live, something to do, and someone to love.'

Somewhere to live

Alex regarded living with his parents as temporary but did not want to return to London. He was uncomfortable with the idea of living alone without something to keep him busy, and he was excruciatingly lonely and yearning for real friendships. His tendency in the past has been to make hasty and impulsive decisions to avoid acute distress, with the result that the decisions often led to yet further difficulties.

On his own, Alex went to view several inappropriate flats or houses and became very discouraged with the house hunt. For example, he viewed a house that was shared by university students, which he captured by telling us about the 'please don't use my toothbrush' note he saw in the bathroom. Clearly, this kind of situation was inappropriate for Alex. We decided to use the Goal Management Framework (GMF) (Duncan, 1986; Robertson, 1996) to help Alex with the practical problem of finding a place to live as well as to work on his executive functioning difficulties with planning, organising and thinking through decisions, instead of his usual emotion-based hasty decision making. He completed a GMF (see Figure 17.2) and was supported in following the steps through to the end. He successfully found a lovely furnished house in a good location near a bus route in Cambridge.

Something to do

We all knew that Alex needed meaningful structured daily occupation to tolerate living alone. His occupational therapist set up another GMF to help Alex consider volunteer opportunities that would truly suit him. Together, they looked on a volunteering website and chose a number of options. Then they evaluated the pros and cons of each one and Alex narrowed the list to a few worthy of further research. He chose an opportunity to volunteer with a museum in Cambridge, a setting suited to his background and interests. He was immediately successful, received compliments from museum visitors, and was warmly received by his new boss, so much so that he increased his working hours to almost full-time. Unfortunately, as Alex grew comfortable and at ease in the museum, others became uncomfortable with his disinhibition and he has had to leave the post. We hope to identify another position, but this time with support to anticipate and avoid such problems in the future.

Goal Management Framework

1. What is my goal?
What am I trying to achieve?

↓

Stop–Think

2. What are all the possible solutions?
Think outside the box!

↓

Stop–Think

3. Weigh up the pros and cons and make a decision
*Think about **all** the choices*

↓

Stop–Think

4. Plan the steps
Think about the sequence and timing
Think about what strategies to use

↓

Stop–Think

5. Do it and review it
Am I still on track? Check the mental blackboard.
Is my solution working?
Was it a success, what went well, what went badly?

↓

Stop–Think

Figure 17.2 Alex's Goal Management Framework. (*Continued*)

Stop–Think: What is the main goal?
Find a place to live

Alternative Solutions	Pros	Cons
Live with partner	Ideal	No partner yet
Live with parents	Easier I get fed and watered Comfortable home Community support Cheap	Being with parents Unable to meet anyone Unable to have occupation It's not a societal norm Lack of friends' support
Live with others	Potential friends Away from parents Cook what I like to eat In a town or city with access to night life	Expense Might not get along with them They might be untidy or unclean Might not be a community
Live alone	Easy to find housing Away from parents Cook what I like to eat In a town or city with access to night life	Easier to be horrible to myself Loneliness

Figure 17.2 (continued)

(*Continued overleaf*)

Stop–Think: What solution have you chosen?
Live alone

Plan:

Step	Achieved? ☑ ✗
Step 1: Choose location – decide between Ely and Cambridge, choose Cambridge	✓
Step 2: Consider desired features – location, price, furnished	✓
Step 3: Contact estate agents in Cambridge	✓
Step 4: View possible places	✓
Step 5: Choose and move	✓

Now review it!
Are things going well? If not, do you need to change your plan?

Figure 17.2 (continued)

Someone to love

While Alex ultimately hopes to meet a life partner, he also wants friendships and social engagement. Now that he was settled in Cambridge and working most days, the social connections followed. Because he is a remarkably personable and outgoing man, Alex has easily made friends. We helped facilitate this earlier on by setting him up on a cooking course. He enjoyed the course, but most important, he met a new friend there with whom he continues to socialise. At the museum, he was taken into the family of the managers, spending social evenings with them and meeting their friends.

Alex's impediments to lasting friendships relate to his disinhibition and tendency to say things before thinking through the consequences. To work on this, he started recording all of his 'Oops Moments', or 'OopMo's' as they became known, on his phone and sending them through as emails for review in his Cognitive and Mood sessions. As Alex's awareness of these moments increased through attending to and recording them, he began to use Stop–Think – literally just stopping and thinking before acting. This helped him retract unsuitable comments before they were made. Most important, these tools helped Alex to have control over his comments to others and reduced his need to apologise.

During parts of his rehabilitation, Alex completed daily ratings of his sense of wellbeing on a scale of 1 to 7, with 1 being suicidal and 5 being an acceptable goal. In the early days, his ratings ranged from just under 2 to 3 or 3.5. By the time he accomplished home and work goals, his ratings have ranged from 4 to 5 and even higher. However, now that he is no longer at the museum, the ratings have dropped again.

The next stage

We considered these goals to be necessary but not sufficient for Alex to feel satisfied with rehabilitation. His fixed and strong beliefs that a positive life was not possible for him and his constant and vicious negative self-talk have been extremely intransigent. We have drawn on elements of Cognitive Behaviour Therapy and Compassion Focused Therapy to help Alex recognise negative thoughts early on, substitute kinder and more compassionate thoughts, and reflect on the difference in mood that comes with thinking kind thoughts. We have also brought in the concept of metacognitive thinking to help Alex zoom out from the immediate moment to see the bigger picture. He is learning not to predict his future from his past (i.e. the belief that things always went wrong before and therefore they always will) and to feel safe with a positive experience in the present. The safety will come once he is able to recognise, monitor and control his own thoughts and actions, and therefore to have predictability in himself and in his future.

Alex's story is ongoing. He has not considered his rehabilitation to be successful because he does not currently have enough meaningful things to do and he remains lonely. His work will be to recognise his accomplishments, plan how to encounter and get through future challenges and, overall, to continue meandering through the delta. At this writing, he has suspended but not ended his rehabilitation with us.

Chapter 18

Karen's story

Putting the pieces back together again

Jill Winegardner and Karen Rich

Karen had everything going for her – a husband she loved, work she enjoyed and good health – when a road traffic accident in 2002 left her with spinal fractures and a brain injury. Within a few years, she lost her job and her marriage, and ended up back home with her parents. To make things even worse, she was diagnosed with chronic fatigue syndrome and fibromyalgia, leaving her in a state of exhaustion. Now, ten years on, inpatient rehab helped her recover some energy, retrieve her independence and gain confidence. At the Oliver Zangwill Centre (OZC) she started putting the pieces of her life back together again.

Introduction

Now 41 years old, Karen grew up in a Lincolnshire town, the daughter of factory workers. Karen's family, including her younger brother, have all stayed settled in Lincolnshire. She described them as preferring to stay settled while she yearned for adventure.

Karen completed school at 16 with average grades, though she was a conscientious and hard-working student, saying that schoolwork did not come easily to her. She then earned a diploma in Hotel Management, earning distinctions. Around that time, though, she met her husband and put her career on hold to be with him. She married at 20 and held a number of jobs, ranging from factory work to working on a cruise ship before starting a career as a flight attendant in 2001. She loved this job and stayed with it until June 2007, but eventually she was unable to cope with it due to fatigue. As we were to learn, there was more to Karen's history than we first knew.

During my childhood and adolescent years, I was exposed to and witnessed many things that I had to deal with. At those times my way of coping was to hide away from my worries, fears, pain, sadness etc. and be strong for and take care of others in the situation. Over the years, unbeknown to me at the time, this became my protection system to try and save myself more suffering. The memories were still there, packed neatly away from daily view, but the concrete was slowly being poured into a mould around my fragile heart, in order to save it any more breakages.

I continued with life and its 'ups and downs' and for most was able to control these 'locked up', negative feelings and memories inside. However, a series of life-changing events, which took place whilst in my thirties, definitely changed that as my defence system became open and exposed once more.

Background of injury

Yes, a trio of events turned life as I'd known it upside down. The first being on 1 August 2002. Whilst driving home from work I was involved in a road traffic accident. Trouble is, that and a period of two weeks was erased from my memory, but to make any sense of it I needed to piece it all together. Well it had happened to me, but without the memories, it was frightening and just didn't seem real.

In hospital Karen was diagnosed with parieto-temporal contusions and seven fractured vertebrae. She had confusion and ten days of post-traumatic amnesia. Karen spent 15 days in hospital before being discharged home in the care of her husband. She received no further treatment other than two physiotherapy visits and checks during the three months post-discharge when she wore a body brace. She received no attention to her brain injury and, in fact, was not even told she had one at that time.

Believing I could return to life as before, I raced towards improvement so I could go back to work and routine as soon as possible. In fact, only four months after my accident I started part-time work for a friend, before continuing at the airline within the year. Unfortunately, around this time my nan became very ill and was diagnosed with terminal colon cancer. Despite this and the fact that she was 97, I had in no way prepared myself for her death. Understandably, when the time came, a few months later, I was terribly upset. However, as the years passed I still grieved deeply as I missed her love. You see, she was the only member of my family who ever told me that she loved me or showed genuine affection towards me. What did I do though? I pushed it aside and just tried to get on with life, which wasn't always as easy as it may have seemed to those around. It's amazing what a smile can hide!

Lastly in the trio of events, and for me almost life-shattering, was the break-down of my marriage. I had been married for 12 years and I couldn't and didn't want to imagine my life without him. I can't even begin to tell you the pain I suffered. I was heartbroken. My whole world felt like it had fallen apart. This time, although I tried for a long time, I was unable to hide it away so easily. It was there every minute of every day and I had no place to hide.

Fortunately, we were able to be civilised and agreeable, but it's only now, almost eight years on, that I can say I've decided to be thankful and embrace being single. Until now, I've been searching for a replacement to give me what I had; the love, compassion, kindness, warmth, gentleness, comfort, courage, strength and confi-dence that I so desperately craved in my life. It's true I became like a woman possessed as I spent six years frantically searching and the only thing I managed to accumulate was a host of health problems. Not exactly what I was looking for.

Until this time, Karen's life revolved around her work, travel and her marriage. In the next few years, she began experiencing exhaustion that made it very difficult for her to maintain work. She decided to take a career break and moved to Latvia teaching English as a volunteer. She found that she was not able to keep up with the requirements and had many sick days. After a year, she asked her parents to come and collect her things and she moved back home with her mother and stepfather in 2008.

By the end of 2008 Karen was not only experiencing exhaustion but was having other physical symptoms and was finally admitted to hospital for two weeks, where she underwent numerous tests, including psychological tests, and was told she had sustained a brain injury in the 2002 accident.

Although Karen first learned she had a brain injury during her hospital admission of 2008, she acknowledged that she has poor memory of the first years post-injury and confined her life to home and work. She recalls experiencing cognitive difficulties from immediately post-injury and these difficulties forced her to work extra hard to get the same results as before and to reduce her activities. Neuropsychological assessment revealed problems with memory, executive function, insight and emotional control. In addition she was diagnosed with chronic fatigue syndrome (CFS).

During 2009 Karen took a job as a teaching assistant but had to reduce her hours over time to a low of six hours a week. Finally, in mid-2010, she had to quit altogether, again due to fatigue and exhaustion.

Karen's relationship with her mother and stepfather suffered during the last couple of years that she lived with them. She described them as telling her to 'just get on with it' and said that tensions mounted between them to the point that she needed to leave in early 2011.

Inpatient rehabilitation

Karen's falling out with her family precipitated an admission to a brain-injury residential programme. Prior to this, she did not shower daily and needed her mother's help to wash her hair due to fatigue. She fixed simple meals and kept her room tidy, but was unable to manage any other household chores. She found shopping difficult due to anxiety about noise and crowds and to problems with decision making. She returned to driving after her accident but initially found it very emotionally challenging. She struggled with finances and had limited participation in social and physical recreational pursuits.

At the residential programme, she was encouraged to participate in more structured routine activities and build physical and mental tolerance. She progressed well with a walking programme and gained independence showering and washing her hair, though still not daily. She moved to an independent living flat as part of the programme, and this gave her the opportunity to test out her abilities in a safe environment. Eventually she regained sufficient independent living skills to live in her own flat while attending the Oliver Zangwill Centre (OZC).

Assessment

Karen first came to the OZC for a two-day Admissions Assessment. She is a small woman with dark curly hair and no physical indications of injury. When we met Karen, we found her to be friendly and communicative, though she appeared timid, shy and anxious initially. She was very soft spoken and tended to provide excess details to answers. She showed a normal range of emotional expression and she interacted well with staff and clients in the centre.

Karen was accepted on to the programme and her assessment was continued during the first few weeks of the programme. Results from the Admissions Assessment and further detailed assessment were combined to yield formulations in each of several key areas that were used to guide her rehabilitation plan.

Physical assessment

Karen described problems with chronic fatigue as well as headaches and pain due to fibromyalgia and irritable bowel syndrome. This meant that fatigue management and pain tolerance would be necessary components of her programme.

Cognitive assessment

Karen reported many cognitive difficulties, including poor concentration and memory, word-finding problems, poor decision-making and problem solving, and trouble initiating, planning and carrying through tasks. She said she tended to 'make odd remarks, tactless comments, and then beat myself up'.

Cognitive testing revealed normal intelligence and memory. Karen showed mild difficulties with speed of information processing, divided attention and aspects of executive functioning including effective strategy choice and planning. It was also clear that her anxiety and lack of confidence played a role in her approach to the tests, as she anticipated a much worse performance than she actually gave.

Functional assessment

Karen's level of functioning within a community setting was assessed during a trip into the local community with instructions to carry out several tasks such as shopping in the supermarket, buying a hot drink and finding options for a gift at the gift shop. She rated her confidence before and after the trip. Her anxiety and low self-confidence were apparent, but she completed the tasks capably with some prompts and reassurance. Again, her self-appraisal was very low and a mismatch with her performance.

Karen was then observed completing a novel computer-based task incorporating accessing information from the internet to attend a social event. The purpose of the task was to assess cognitive abilities such as attention, planning and organisation on a real-life functional task. Again her confidence ratings were very low and under-rated her ability. As with the community outing, she required cueing and prompts as well as reassurance to manage anxiety. Challenges were noted in attention and strategy use.

Assessment tools from the Model of Human Occupation (MOHO) (Kielhofner, Braveman, Baron, Fisher, Hammel & Littleton, 1999) were used to explore Karen's motivation, values and interests. Karen was uncertain about her desired occupational identity and repeatedly stated that she felt lost, overwhelmed and as if she did not know who she is or what she wants. She had several interests and strongly held values, which would be important to consider in establishing her future occupational identity, especially her Christian faith and creativity. Although she engaged in a range of activities, she reported reduced satisfaction with all tasks. Karen attempted to pace herself by building in breaks, but did not rest effectively as she found it difficult to switch off mentally. Developing strategies to support relaxation was therefore identified as a key goal. Her occupational formulation is found in Figure 18.1.

Mood assessment

Karen talked of difficulties with anxiety, intense feelings of anger and angry outbursts, low mood and passive suicidal ideation. She experienced a negative impact of chronic fatigue syndrome on her mood, as well as loss of pleasure, lack of confidence and a lack of closeness in family relationships. At the start of her rehabilitation programme she also reported difficulties with her sense of being able to achieve what she sets out to do (self-efficacy), either thinking of herself as a 'failure' who 'can't live up to expectations' or thinking of herself as being 'able to do anything' and doing too much, then feeling overwhelmed.

I came to the OZC with more baggage than I like to think about and no I don't mean holdalls, I mean emotional baggage. 'Where did it all come from?', you may be thinking, as I know I certainly was.

Karen had suffered multiple losses in recent years that she struggled to accept. Her acquired brain injury, combined with fibromyalgia and CFS, had resulted in further changes and multiple losses (of friendships, employment, leisure activities, valued roles), which had reactivated memories of other losses and triggered a long period of anxiety and low mood, maintained by an avoidant coping style and losses as a result of the brain injury. Karen's behaviour also suggested that she has struggled to manage to cope independently and coped by becoming dependent on others, which also played a role in maintaining avoidance and lack of confidence and her lack of sense of agency.

Communication assessment

Karen's communication goal was to establish herself socially in her new town. Our assessment of her social communication skills revealed only mild difficulty with recognising the emotions of sadness, anger and anxiety as well as in picking up on sarcasm. The results did not match with Karen's very negative self-report on questionnaires nor with observations of her in the centre. Instead, she was seen to be functioning at a very high level, but her performance was heavily impacted by her state of

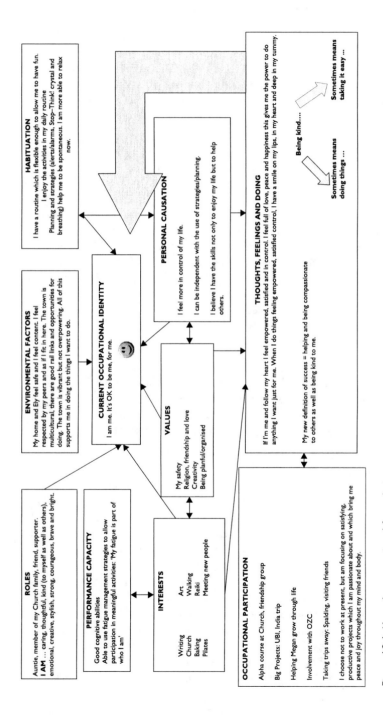

ROLES
Auntie, member of my Church family, friend, supporter.
I AM ... caring, thoughtful, kind (to myself as well as others), emotional, creative, stylish, strong, courageous, brave and bright.

ENVIRONMENTAL FACTORS
My home and Ely feel safe and I feel content. I feel respected by my peers and as if I fit in here. The town is multicultural, there are good rail links and opportunities for doing. The town is vibrant but not overpowering. All of this supports me in doing the things I want to do.

HABITUATION
I have a routine which is flexible enough to allow me to have fun. I enjoy the activities in my daily routine. Planning and strategies (alerts/alarms, Stop–Think! crystal and breathing) help me to be spontaneous. I am more able to relax now.

PERFORMANCE CAPACITY
Good cognitive abilities
Able to use fatigue management strategies to allow participation in meaningful activities: 'My fatigue is part of who I am'

CURRENT OCCUPATIONAL IDENTITY
I am me. It's OK to be me, for me.

PERSONAL CAUSATION
I feel more in control of my life.
I can be independent with the use of strategies/planning.
I believe I have the skills not only to enjoy my life but to help others.

VALUES
My safety
Religion, friendship and love
Creativity
Being planful/organised

INTERESTS
Writing   Art
Church   Walking
Baking   Reiki
Pilates   Meeting new people

THOUGHTS, FEELINGS AND DOING
If I'm me and follow my heart I feel empowered, satisfied and in control. I feel full of love, peace and happiness this gives me the power to do anything I want just for me. When I do things feeling empowered, satisfied control, I have a smile on my lips, in my heart and deep in my tummy.

My new definition of success = helping and being compassionate to others as well as being kind to me.

Being kind....

Sometimes means doing things ...

Sometimes means taking it easy ...

OCCUPATIONAL PARTICIPATION
Alpha course at Church, friendship group
Big Projects: UBI, India trip
Helping Megan grow through life
Involvement with OZC
Taking trips away: Spalding, visiting friends
I choose not to work at present, but am focusing on satisfying, productive projects which I am passionate about and which bring me peace and joy throughout my mind and body.

Figure 18.1 Karen's occupational formulation.

mind, i.e. mood, fatigue and high expectations of herself. In addition, Karen was observed to have many strengths, such as good verbal reasoning, good discourse ability including word-finding, a good sense of humour and an assertive style. The latter was not easily acknowledged as she did not feel confident, although this was not always apparent to the observer.

Rehabilitation

Karen's goals on entering the programme were to understand her brain injury, to receive help for emotional trauma, to set herself up to return to community life and to cope better with life's challenges. She wanted to 'find out who I am and where I fit in life' and to regain confidence. Together we set up several rehabilitation goals.

So there I was, nine years later, at OZC ready to start my rehab programme. It was intensive, but it gave me an excellent framework. So when it came to my individual sessions the language wasn't all alien. Well not all of it anyway!

With the team's support, Karen set herself ambitious goals.

Goal 1: Karen will gain an understanding of the nature and consequences of her brain injury and learn strategies to manage her difficulties with cognition, communication, mood and fatigue

Karen participated actively in the psycho-education course and acquired good basic knowledge of brain injury overall, as well as an understanding of how each key area (attention and memory, executive functions, communication and mood) is affected by brain injury in general and her injury in particular. Karen had the opportunity to review and understand the medical notes and scans from the time of her injury, and to put together a timeline of key events from this stage in her recovery.

During those sessions I had access to my hospital records and scans. The team worked through them with me so I could build a better picture of what had happened. For the first time, I felt I could ask questions about my injuries without feeling 'stupid' or worrying that I should already know the answer. No, the team at OZC went at my pace (once we'd found a more suitable one for my fatigue) and were a wealth of knowledge. At the same time they made me feel safe and not alone, which was hugely comforting for me.

Goal 2: Karen will learn mindfulness as a strategy to improve both attention and mood

We decided that Detached Mindfulness (Kabat-Zinn, 2005) would be a useful technique to develop control over Karen's attention system and would also complement her mood work. We taught her the principles of mindfulness and how to use a mindfulness meditation CD for practice.

Karen achieved this goal and demonstrated commitment to engaging in mindfulness practice. She reported increased metacognitive control as a consequence of engaging in mindfulness. She explained that she is now much more frequently aware of her negative automatic thoughts as they arise and their accompanied emotions and can ground her attention to her present experience. This has a number of consequences: it allows her to remove herself from getting caught up in cycles of rumination, and it reduces the emotional impact of these cycles. She also described improved performance and greater satisfaction in her daily tasks. She began engaging in mindfulness in everyday activities, where she focused her attention to one element of the task that she is doing in order to anchor her attention to her current experience. She described that this has altered her experience of these tasks and helped her to tolerate uncomfortable feelings.

Goal 3: Karen will learn fatigue management as well as gain satisfaction and confidence in her activities

Although Karen was engaging in a reasonable level of occupational activity at the beginning of the programme, she reported an absence of satisfaction with all tasks, as well as a loss of sense of self. Her fatigue, tendency towards perfectionism and desire to please other people contributed significantly to this loss of enjoyment.

The first stage of the intervention involved supporting fatigue management and enhancing Karen's sense of control through planning and pacing. She chose to trial a Filofax, and engaged extremely well with this tool, developing her own systems for planning activity, keeping track of tasks she needs to do, noting down ideas to pursue in the future and maintaining a success log. She now uses the Filofax consistently and independently, and reports finding it helpful.

Work on fatigue management also involved trialling activities to help Karen relax effectively. These included soothing breathing, mindful bubble baths and taking short breaks every ten minutes during periods of intense activity. Karen has also identified that, on occasion, engaging with a pleasurable activity can help her to relax and self-soothe. During a particularly challenging period when Karen was tending to ruminate excessively, she found it helpful to take a break from 'talking' sessions and to focus instead on an enjoyable practical task (baking).

Following these experiments, Karen initiated, planned, carried out and reported enjoying a number of activities with minimal support. By the end of the programme, she felt sufficiently confident in using her strategies to apply them to a task that she had previously found extremely challenging (internet shopping). Karen's strategies were summarised in the form of a set of 'recipes' to which she can refer in a range of situations.

The progress made by Karen during the programme is reflected in the positive change in scores for the Canadian Occupational Performance Measure (COPM) (Law et al., 1990), which was applied at the beginning and the end of the programme. Particular improvement was noted in her ratings for satisfaction. Notable changes were observed in personal causation, occupational participation and habituation, which in turn impact positively on Karen's thoughts, feelings and engagement with occupation.

Goal 4: Karen will learn to be compassionate to herself

Key techniques developed to achieve the goal were taken from Compassionate Mind Training (CMT) (Gilbert, 2005, 2010a, 2010b): soothing rhythm breathing, safe-place imagery, compassionate other imagery, compassionate letter writing, compassionate self-imagery and mindfulness. Psycho-education was also provided about panic disorder. Karen was encouraged to regularly practise these exercises despite struggles to engage her soothing system. A key part of our work was helping her acknowledge and address fears and blocks towards self-compassion. For Karen there were clear barriers, rooted in her pre-injury experiences; these were addressed through compassionate letter writing, which encourages understanding and tolerance of one's own distress.

Towards the end of the programme, Karen described feeling a much stronger response from her soothing system when she self-soothed or engaged in CMT. She described being able to pause when she notices her threat system being activated and to choose to react to the situation from her soothing system with a more compassionate approach. This was reflected in the outcome measurement questionnaires as her scores

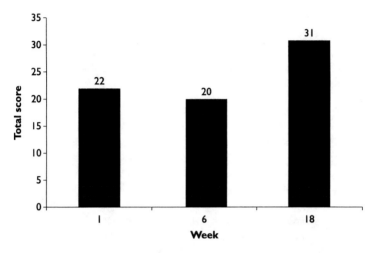

Figure 18.2 General self-efficacy scale from week 1 to week 18 of the programme.

reflecting her ability to reassure herself increased significantly, and scores relating to self-criticism (inadequate and hated self) reduced significantly. Accordingly, her self-esteem rose and her experience of depression and anxiety is now reported to be mild.

At every turn I learned and continue to learn something new about myself. The whole experience is quite liberating and immensely satisfying, as I open and slowly empty my emotional baggage.

Next to this lies my vanity case, which travels everywhere with me. If you took a peek inside you'd see my constant, chronic fatigue. Yes, it soon became evident that to better manage my fatigue, I'd have to somehow reduce the constant threat in my life and try to find my own self-soothing system. Now this whole being kind and compassionate to myself was new ground for me and took a while to adjust to.

We did many experiments and tried many strategies before I finally found my great new tool kit. Now that really is infallible. With my prayers, Filofax, my phone alerts, my soothing breathing and compassionate writing I can weather most emotional storms given time. A huge improvement I never thought I would ever see.

Don't get me wrong, by no means am I perfect. I still try to hide away and avoid things that are difficult to face up to, but the difference is now I am conscious of what I am doing. Then it's up to me if, what, when, where, why, who and how I deal with it. Not as easy as it sounds I admit, but it's all progress.

Goal 5: Karen will increase both her participation and her confidence and satisfaction in social activity

Karen wanted to explore various social activities in the community to build her confidence and also to challenge negative beliefs about herself through the process. A graded hierarchy of social activities was developed. Each step on her hierarchy was treated as a behavioural experiment. Karen completed an experiments sheet prior to carrying the experiment out, noting her predictions and any planned strategies she was using. These strategies included both cognitive strategies such as the Goal Management Framework (Duncan, 1986; Robertson, 1996) to brainstorm options and the 5 Ws and H (who/what/where/when/why and how) to focus her planning, along with mood strategies, such as relaxation techniques. Karen reflected on each experiment and noted what actually happened, with objective feedback (video playback) being sought where possible. She then discussed with her therapist her reflections on strategies used and the impact on her identity.

Karen also developed a number of strategies to build her social confidence, including taking up Reiki sessions again, making time for herself, pacing, managing her diet, using alerts to ensure taking time out and using her attention beam. As the last step in the hierarchy, Karen successfully read her own poetry at a Cambridge open mic event. Karen's confidence and satisfaction both rose significantly after she achieved all the steps in her hierarchy.

UBI project

As part of her rehabilitation, Karen undertook a UBI (Understanding Brain Injury) project to depict her journey through her injury and her rehabilitation. She created a collage reflecting her life from infancy through today, using many different artistic media.

Throughout my sessions I kept notes, but there was so much for me to process in my own time. Therefore, it was only after the programme finished that I found the time, space and energy to start work on my UBI project.

I've been shown I have a purpose in life and I continue to find healing, this time through my UBI project. I will take the difficult journey back through the pain, hurt and sadness in my life and look at it with 'new eyes'. Finding compassion and forgiveness is key to overcoming the blame, shame and guilt that has marred my life. With the skills I've learnt, the support I receive and my faith, I know it is achievable.

By the programme's end, Karen had surpassed the goals she set for herself and had an active social life that was more in keeping with her identity and personality. She organised her social calendar for the next three months and included regular social events, Pilates classes and Friendship group meetings through her church.

In summary, Karen accomplished all goals, including education about brain injury, learning and use of compensatory strategies, and successful implementation of these strategies in key areas of her everyday life and her relationships. The results of the European Brain Injury Questionnaire (EBIQ) and the Dysexecutive Questionnaire (DEX) reflected a decrease in the experience of challenges faced after brain injury by Karen and her family.

With the team's support she developed her own personal toolbox of strategies to overcome the brain-injury related challenges she faces. She has taken ownership of this process and has incorporated these into personal 'recipe cards' that she carries within her Filofax. She has been

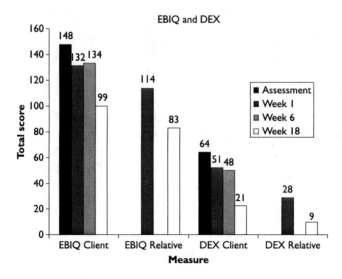

Figure 18.3 European Brain Injury Questionnaire (EBIQ) and the DEX symptom checklist from assessment through to week 18 of the programme.

considerably committed to the rehabilitation process and demonstrated tenacity throughout.

Karen has returned to the OZC for routine reviews throughout her first year post-programme, each time reviewing her progress and setting new goals for herself. She has been highly successful and even completed a mission to India with her church, something that would have been inconceivable prior to rehabilitation. She recently held a celebration of surviving ten years of brain injury with friends and supporters, including OZC staff. Her UBI collage was on display, covering three tables. Karen spoke with amazing confidence and self-assurance about her painful and yet ultimately successful journey through many difficult years, reading a poem she had written that expressed this journey very eloquently.

2012 and this was a year of new beginnings for me. I am starting to look at me and my life through newly focused, self-compassionate eyes. I want to take the fear that has trapped and consumed me and change it into joy and peace, so I can enjoy my life and use some of the amazing gifts I see I've been given.

Last year, 2011, was a big year for me as I turned 40, started brain-injury rehabilitation at the Oliver Zangwill Centre and was reconnected with my faith. Therefore, the positivity, the motivation and determination I gained has spurred me forward onto this project of 'New Beginnings – My Story'.

I never thought or even imagined I'd get such a fantastic opportunity to work alongside the professionals at Oliver Zangwill for my rehab. Nevertheless, here I am after completing my programme and writing to tell you guys about my story. It's a slow process to uncover all of those things but a combination of my faith and the OZC has shown me it's all there inside of me. It's just waiting and wanting to be nurtured. Unfortunately, the disappointing news for me seems to be there's no quick fix or magic cure. It will take time and patience to heal these deep, emotional wounds of the past. However, I'm now heading in the right, albeit new, direction on my journey.

Hopefully in the future I can help others who have found themselves in similar situations. An important thing to remember is hope. On my journey I've learned no matter how insurmountable life seems, always have hope.

'Out of my darkness, I have found gold.'

Chapter 19

Concluding remarks

Barbara A. Wilson and Jill Winegardner

We have presented a series of stories of men and women whose normal lives were dramatically interrupted by illness or injury to the brain. Their injuries ranged from so-called mild post-concussive syndrome to the profound locked-in syndrome. For all of them, the injuries drastically altered their lives and for most of them life has not returned to pre-injury 'normality'. All have engaged in a journey of rehabilitation that has led them to a new adjustment, a new understanding and appreciation of the possibilities of life and their own potential to come to peace with their new selves.

As clinicians in an increasingly impoverished health-care climate, we know our rehabilitation resources are limited and precious. It is urgent that we identify the characteristics of the people who are most likely to benefit from rehabilitation, so that those most likely to benefit are the ones offered the service.

What then are key characteristics of the people featured in this book that have allowed them to rise to the rehabilitation challenge so effectively? What differentiates them from those clients with similar injuries whose outcomes were not positive? We must examine several factors: characteristics of the clients themselves; the nature of their injuries; the nature and quality of the rehabilitation; and the right match of type of rehabilitation to client.

In reflecting on these clients, as well as on those who have not fared so well in rehabilitation, we consider factors that differentiate responders from non-responders. The people represented in this book shared a number of features that have been shown to correlate with positive outcomes in rehabilitation, such as the following:

• at least a minimum level of awareness and insight;

- expectations for rehabilitation that roughly match the clinician's expectations (these may be culturally mediated);
- no serious history of pre-injury psychological disorders;
- absence of drug and alcohol abuse;
- presence of family support;
- availability of local resources (health, vocational, social services);
- a minimum level of socioeconomic security;
- good engagement with rehabilitation services from the onset;
- personality qualities and traits including determination.

Even so, these features were not necessarily found in everyone, but their presence certainly enhanced the therapeutic process.

We also consider whether there is something about the nature of the injury that influences the eventual level of success of rehabilitation. We have seen in this series that severity of injury is not a conclusive determinant, with good outcomes possible regardless of injury severity. Perhaps the key here is the appropriateness of the goals that are set and the acceptance of these goals by both client and therapist.

In previous work describing holistic neuropsychological rehabilitation, the core components considered necessary to enable successful rehabilitation have been listed. They have been illustrated in this book, for example: (i) successfully working with families or the wider system; (ii) focusing on meaningful functional activity; (iii) finding the right compensatory strategy that can help overcome communication, cognitive or emotional impairments; (iv) providing therapy within a safe therapeutic milieu; (v) providing appropriate models of psychological therapy; and (vi) having an effective approach to sharing our understanding of the client within the interdisciplinary team and the wider system.

The survivors' stories indicate that a meaningful life is possible despite brain injury, which in some cases is obviously severe. There may be persisting cognitive, emotional and sometimes physical problems and, occasionally, there may have been long periods of limited responsiveness. Some of the survivors are several years post-injury or illness and it is evident that this should not be considered a barrier to rehabilitation. Many of them experienced severe fatigue, which is becoming increasingly recognised as a consequence of brain injury and requires specific treatment that needs to be incorporated into rehabilitation programmes. The holistic approach is considered to be crucial for successful rehabilitation in most cases described here. Some of our more profoundly injured survivors did not undergo holistic rehabilitation but they did get the right approach for them. In all cases, the approach was chosen based on a deep understanding of holistic principles.

An apparently mild traumatic brain injury left Tim, an intelligent man, with cognitive and emotional problems severe enough for him to consider suicide and to fill him with doubts about his self-worth. He responded well to the rehabilitation programme and was able to return to work. One of the main messages from Tim's story is that a seemingly trivial injury can cause major problems and that this is not always recognised by the medical profession. Neuropsychologists, too, can miss the genuine difficulties faced by people after what appear to be superficial accidents. The holistic approach, including a safe milieu, is shown to be effective in dealing with the cognitive and emotional consequences of Tim's 'mild' traumatic brain injury (TBI).

Having suffered a subarachnoid haemorrhage at the age of 24 years, Natalie managed to return to work for a number of years despite fatigue and epilepsy. She was eventually referred to the OZC at the age of 32 years. She attended for an assessment but her health authority would not, initially, fund the holistic programme. Things became worse and Natalie attempted suicide. Eventually, funding was obtained for her to attend the intensive, comprehensive holistic programme. Natalie, whose artwork appears on the frontispiece of this book, now works as a pet portraitist and is also an ambassador for a mental health trust. From Natalie's story we learn that refusing funding can lead to even more expensive costs at the end of the day. When there was no consistent and targeted rehabilitation Natalie made a suicide attempt and required health-care input, which might have been avoided had her needs been addressed properly earlier on (Winegardner & Ashworth, 2012).

Twelve years after a severe TBI, Eliot was referred for rehabilitation. He had considerable problems with executive deficits. Until fairly recently these were considered to be resistant to rehabilitation. Goal management training (Robertson, 1996 and Levine *et al.*, 2000), based on Duncan's (1986) model of goal neglect, together with Problem Solving Training (e.g Von Cramon *et al.*, 1991) has changed the situation, however, and now we have some very successful results (e.g. Miotto *et al.*, 2009). Eliot responded well to his rehabilitation programme. His passion for golf was a key to motivating him and much of his treatment focused around his chosen sport. Eliot's story is persuasive in encouraging therapists to incorporate the individual's personal interests and lifestyle into any programme as far as possible.

Kate was not able to participate in a milieu-based programme, but her assessment was key to her recovery. Her story shows that recovery can continue for many years, despite several months of very limited responsiveness when she first became ill with acute disseminated encephalomyelitis. Kate was considered to be intellectually impaired until she had a detailed neuropsychological assessment two years post-illness. She received neuropsychological treatment for more than eight years and this, together with her own determination and strong personality, allowed her to pull through to a stage where she now lives in her own specially built bungalow.

A successful student, Jose David's medical studies came to an end as a result of hypoxic brain damage sustained in a routine operation to remove cartilage in his knee. The main focus of Jose David's story is his introduction to a memory strategy that enabled him to return to study again. He retrained as a medical anthropologist and now works for the government in his country, Colombia. He continues to use a modified version of this strategy in his everyday life.

Despite having locked-in syndrome (LIS), which means she is intellectually intact but completely paralysed apart from being able to move her eyes, Tracey feels she has a reasonable quality of life and engages well with the world. She illustrates the view of Laureys *et al.* (2005) that although most able-bodied and healthy people think that life with LIS would not be worth living, most people with LIS do not feel this. People tend to assume there is an intellectual deficit for people with severe physical handicaps but Tracey, like Kate, had average or above average intellectual functioning, highlighting the importance of appropriate neuropsychological assessment.

A motorcycle accident caused James's TBI. He agreed to go to the OZC for rehabilitation but initially found it difficult to engage. The staff spent some time building up a good rapport and eventually James recognised the need to participate fully. Most clients at the OZC are encouraged to build a portfolio to help understand what happened to cause the brain injury and subsequent problems. In James's case this involved reviewing his medical records and physiotherapy notes to help him piece together events surrounding and immediately after his accident, and also to challenge some unhelpful beliefs he had formed. Like Eliot's passion for golf, James's skill at drawing was employed to help him through the rehabilitation programme. He was able, through drawings, to indicate what had happened to him and illustrate visually some of his emotions. His severe depression was treated jointly by the neuropsychologist and a neuropsychiatrist. James's story indicates how important it is to initially allow time to build up a rapport and include other therapies when necessary: in his case, joint work with a neuropsychiatrist and psychological therapy that incorporated his art.

Following herpes simplex viral encephalitis, Claire was left with considerable emotional and cognitive difficulties, the main one being prosopagnosia, a failure to recognise faces. Claire's insights and her ability to portray her feelings in a clear and coherent writing style provide us with a poignant and moving insider's view of this huge handicap. Her story also illustrates the value of the rehabilitation Claire received for her emotional as well as her cognitive problems and her own willingness to engage and profit from the process.

At the age of 34 years, Jason suffered three strokes within 48 hours. He had a right posterior artery stroke that left him with Wallenberg Syndrome in which there is a loss of pain and temperature sensation on the *contralateral* (opposite) side of the body and *ipsilateral* (same) side of the face. Like other survivors we have described, Jason attempted to return to work and failed. Similarly also, he had both cognitive and emotional problems – particularly with low self-esteem, depression and anxiety. Jason had been a carpenter and joiner prior to his strokes and, as we saw with Eliot and James, he used what he was good at to understand some of his problems. In Jason's case he made a model of the brain from wood to help him understand his brain damage. He also had problems with sleep. This is not uncommon following damage to the brain but it is often under-investigated and under-treated. We learn from Jason's experiences in rehabilitation that accompanying problems such as sleep should always be investigated and treated.

For over two years after being diagnosed with tuberculous meningitis, Christine remained little more than minimally conscious. Yet, one day, she suddenly woke up and gradually improved over the next few months. She still has significant problems but is sociable and chatty and enjoys painting and going on outings. Her story shows how difficult it can be to obtain the right diagnosis (she was thought at one stage to be suffering from anorexia nervosa). Eventual successful treatment illustrates how we should not stop trying to aim for better functioning. From being mute and stuporous, Christine became a fully engaged member of society.

A successful, hard-working engineer, Adrian sustained multiple injuries in a road traffic accident and came to the OZC a year later. He thought he was beyond help, but gradually he engaged with the programme and things went well. Sometime following his discharge, however, his wife divorced him and Adrian deteriorated to the extent that he became severely depressed. Because he trusted the staff at the OZC he was referred to us once more. Again, rehabilitation was successful for Adrian who now has a fulfilling, happy life. One of the main points to emerge from Adrian's story is that some people need a 'top up' or 'booster' dose of rehabilitation when life's circumstances change.

Although Lorraine appeared to be fully conscious after a road traffic accident at the age of 50, she suffered a hypoxic brain injury as a result of the damage to her lungs. Highly anxious with post-traumatic stress disorder, Lorraine wanted to understand what was wrong with her as she could not make sense of the consequences of her injury. Two messages are highlighted in this story. First is the importance of participating in a group because this gives participants an opportunity to support and learn from each other. Second is the importance of working together with families: family support and education were provided for Lorraine's daughter, son and best friend. It is also worth noting that Lorraine, herself, believes that what really helped was being able to understand why she was the way she was after the accident.

Despite sustaining a severe traumatic brain injury after falling 1,000 feet down a mountain in Switzerland, Mark is one of those rare people who has been able to return to and retain a high-powered job. He has been so successful that in the past year he has been headhunted for four senior posts. Since rehabilitation he is happily married with two daughters. His is surely a good outcome in anybody's book! Mark recognises that without rehabilitation, he would have returned to work too soon, almost certainly failed and then been labelled as unemployable. Through his rehabilitation, Mark was able to recognise his difficulties, find ways to deal with them, engage in a gradual return to employment and become the successful man he is today.

Like Mark, Jose David has a successful career, and few would suspect he had survived a serious brain injury. Those survivors who do as well as Mark and Jose David may well succeed because of cognitive reserve. The principle of cognitive reserve says that people with more education and high intelligence may show less impairment than those with poor education and low intelligence. Stern (2007) suggests that individuals with high intelligence may process tasks in a more efficient way. We would suggest that in addition to cognitive reserve, one needs intact frontal lobes to be able to return to demanding jobs.

At the age of 20 years, Vicky was involved in a car accident and sustained a severe TBI. Like some of the other survivors, Vicky returned to work where she struggled to cope, suffered from fatigue and had poor self-esteem. These are all common themes in many of our survivors' stories. Although she lived in Jersey, Vicky was referred to the OZC in Cambridgeshire and, fortunately, her boyfriend moved to Ely with her for the six-month programme. The OZC clients start the programme in cohorts and Vicky's was the first time that the cohort consisted of women only. This seemed to be a positive thing for her and gender-specific issues could be addressed openly. From Vicky's story we realise that when people are attending a centre many miles from their home town, care needs to be taken to ensure that appropriate accommodation is found. Many health authorities take the view that all patients should be treated within their own catchment area but highly specialised services, such as the OZC, are not to be found in every health authority. It is therefore sometimes necessary for survivors of brain injury to be treated by non-local expert services where appropriate accommodation must be provided.

A cerebellar stroke meant Robert had few cognitive difficulties but suffered from severe fatigue and was hyper sensitive to noise. He had good physiotherapy early on after his stroke but little help with the psychological consequences. Fortunately, he was referred to and accepted on the OZC rehabilitation programme. He found the psychological therapy and strategies for dealing with fatigue valuable. What we learn from Robert's story is the importance of explanation to the survivor of a brain injury. Robert did not expect or understand the less common consequences of his stroke and responded well when given appropriate explanations. He found the detailed feedback on his brain scan particularly reassuring and carried around a photo of his scan in his pocket to remind himself of what had occurred and to explain to others what had happened to him.

Unlike others in this book, Alex did not have the rehabilitation outcome he had hoped for. We would agree with Alex that certain aspects of his programme did not go as planned and this contributed to a disappointing experience. In addition, Alex recognised that his fundamental challenge was acceptance of his injury and its implications for his life. Alex believed that acceptance would mean lesser quality of life, and he resisted it. As a result, he did not fully embrace the strategies recommended to him by the team and did not experience the reduction in discrepancy between his pre-injury and his post-injury self that is so essential for coming to grips with such a catastrophic event.

Following a road traffic accident, Karen sustained a TBI although she was not told she had a brain injury until several years later. Her natural shyness, low self-confidence and reluctance to accept her limitations interacted with the cognitive difficulties and were compounded by chronic fatigue syndrome. Karen had many strengths and a good level of functioning, but her mood, fatigue and high expectations of herself meant she did not acknowledge her strengths. One of the main messages illustrated by Karen's story and the rehabilitation given to her is that it is important to proceed at a pace suitable for each individual person: therapists must find the most appropriate strategies for each individual to manage their difficulties and encourage them to be compassionate to themselves.

As was indicated earlier, rehabilitation for individuals with brain injury can be successful, given the right circumstances and family and community support in combination with professional expertise. It is hoped that the stories in this book bear adequate witness to this. In future we should be able to observe a growing awareness in society of the problems faced by brain-injured individuals and a developing understanding of the means to overcome or circumnavigate some of them. This, as always, will result from scientific research and an ensuing development of professional expertise in treatment. Again, it is hoped that this book has taken a few steps in this direction. If the political will were there, and politicians could see the economic benefits to be gained from rehabilitation therapy, such treatment could be provided on a scale that would ensure that all who needed it could benefit to varying degrees, wherever they lived and whatever their financial circumstances. Personal, familial, communal and economic goals must be targeted in order to bring down costs and free people with brain injuries, as far as possible, from some of their disabling and burdensome problems that ultimately affect the well-being of society as a whole. Barbara Wilson's framework for action, described in the first chapter, provides guidance through the maze of considerations that will need to be taken on board if progress is to be made.

With this framework the therapists who have described their work in this book have tied their intentions to the mast, and it is up to the reader to decide whether the diagnoses and treatment described in later pages have been conducted in accordance, as far as possible, with the structure it provides. Obviously, the model is applicable in a *general* sense to all clients but not all parts of the model apply specifically to each individual because in some cases particular areas are implied or are not relevant. Nevertheless, the reader can reflect on the following questions and consider whether, in general or in part, the model has been adhered to in the treatment programmes described:

- Most importantly, have the subsequent daily lives of the clients been improved to any extent by the professional practice described, and does this in any way reflect the therapist's attention to current neuropsychological theory?

- Was the pre-morbid personality and lifestyle of the client considered?
- Were personality assessments and family and community opinions taken into account?
- Were the clients' cognitive, emotional, psychosocial and behavioural strengths and weaknesses examined and discussed wherever possible with the brain-injured individual and his or her closest friends and family?
- Was any evidence of natural recovery considered and taken into account when treatment was designed?
- Was re-assessment provided and did it include ecologically valid measurement, psychometry, localisation, cognition and exclusion models?
- And did these include language, attention, memory and executive functioning?
- Were emotional models and other psychological therapies included in diagnoses and treatment?
- Were observations of behaviour in both natural and simulated settings conducted and were questionnaires, checklists and rating scales employed in these tasks?
- Were treatment decisions negotiated with the client, family and staff?
- In which areas did treatment focus: impairment, disability or handicap?
- How were theories of learning engaged when teaching clients?
- Was lost function concentrated on or was anatomical reorganisation encouraged?
- Were residual skills employed effectively or were alternative means found?
- Or was the environment modified in any way to ease potential difficulties?
- Was any evidence found to indicate success and how was success evaluated?
- Finally, after evaluation, were approaches to rehabilitation revised where suggested?

The reader is asked to reflect on these questions in the light of the stories told by both the therapists and the clients. In this book we have presented a unique balance of clinical overview and client report. We hope to have given a voice to these people and to have brought their humanity to these pages: they are not simply case studies. Their stories could be any of ours.

References

Allain, P., Joseph, P.A., Isambert, J.L., Le Gall, D. & Emile, J. (1998). Cognitive functions in chronic locked-in syndrome: a report of two cases. *Cortex: A Journal Devoted to the Study of the Nervous System and Behavior*. September, *34*(4), 629–634.

Anderson, C., Dillon, C. & Burns, R. (1993). Life-sustaining treatment and locked-in syndrome. *Lancet, 342*, 867–868.

Arts, W.F., van Dongen, H.R. & Meulstee, J. (1988). Unexpected improvement after prolonged post-traumatic vegetative state. *Acta Neurochirurgica Suppl* (Wien), *44*, 78–79.

Ashworth, F., Clarke, A. & Corfield, J. (2012). Learning to be compassionate to my tricky brain. Poster presented at the international conference of the International Brain Injury Association in Edinburgh, Scotland.

Ashworth, F., Gracey, F. & Gilbert, P. (2011). Compassion Focused Therapy after traumatic brain injury: Theoretical foundations and a case illustration. *Brain Impairment, 12*(2), 128–139.

Baddeley, A.D. (1993). A theory of rehabilitation without a model of learning is a vehicle without an engine: A comment on Caramazza and Hillis. *Neuropsychological Rehabilitation, 3*, 235–244.

Bagby, M.R., Parker, J.D. & Taylor, G.J. (1994). The twenty-item Toronto Alexithymia scale—I. Item selection and cross-validation of the factor structure. *Journal of Psychosomatic Research, 38*(1), 23–32.

Bainbridge, K. (2006). *Kate's story*. Nottingham: Headway.

Bateman, A., Greenfield, E., Evans, J.J. & Wilson, B.A. (2007). Development of a Questionnaire to Assess Experience of Divided Attention Difficulties: Insights Gained from Rasch Analysis. *Brain Impairment*. Abstracts of the meeting of the 4th Symposium on Neuropsychological Rehabilitation. San Sebastian, July 2007.

Bauby J. (1997). *The diving bell and the butterfly* (original title: *Le scaphandre et le papillon*. Robert Laffont: Paris). New York: Knopf.

Ben-Yishay, Y. (1978). *Working approaches to the remediation of cognitive deficits in brain damaged persons. Rehabilitation Monograph No. 59.* New York: New York Medical Center.

Ben-Yishay, Y. (1996). Reflections on the evolution of the therapeutic milieu concept. *Neuropsychological Rehabilitation*, 6(4), 327–343.

Ben-Yishay, Y. (2000). Post acute neuropsychological rehabilitation: a holistic perspective. In A.L. Christensen and B. Uzzell (eds), *International handbook of neuropsychological rehabilitation*. New York: Kluwer Academic/Plenum Publishers.

Ben-Yishay, Y. & Prigatano, G.P. (1990). Cognitive remediation. In M. Rosenthal, E.R. Griffith, M.R. Bond and J.D. Miller (eds), *Rehabilitation of the adult and child with traumatic brain injury* (2nd edn.), pp. 393–409. Philadelphia, PA: F.A. Davis.

Bennett-Levy, J., Westbrook, D., Fennell, M., Cooper, M., Rouf, K. & Hackmann, A. (2004). Behavioural experiments: Historical and conceptual underpinnings. In J. Bennett-Levy, G. Butler, M.J.V. Fennell, A. Hackmann, M. Mueller and D. Westbrook (eds), *The Oxford guide to behavioural experiments in cognitive therapy* (pp. 1–20). Oxford: Oxford University Press.

Blackmore, T.K., Manning, L., Taylor, W.J. & Wallis, R.S. (2008). Therapeutic use of infliximab in tuberculosis to control severe paradoxical reaction of the brain and lymph nodes. *Clinical Infectious Diseases*, 47(10), 83–85.

Burgess, P.W., Alderman, N., Emslie, H., Evans, J.J. & Wilson, B.A. (1996). The dysexecutive questionnaire. In B.A. Wilson, N. Alderman, P.W. Burgess, H. Emslie and J.J. Evans (eds), *Behavioural assessment of the dysexecutive syndrome*. Bury St Edmunds, UK: Thames Valley Test Company.

Chisholm, N. & Gillett, G. (2005). The patient's journey: Living with locked-in syndrome. *British Medical Journal* (Clinical Research Ed.). July 9, 331(7508), 94–97.

Cicerone, K.D., Dahlberg, C., Malec, J.F., Langenbahn, D.M., Felicetti, T., Kneipp, S., Ellmo, W., Kalmar, K., Giacino, J.T., Preston Harley, J., Laatsch, L., Morse, P. & Catanese, J. (2005). Evidence-based cognitive rehabilitation: Updated review of the literature from 1998 through 2002. *Archives of Physical and Medical Rehabilitation*, 86, 1681–1692.

Cicerone, K.D., Langenbahn, D.M, Braden, C., Malec, J.F., Bergquist, T., Azulay, J., Cantor, J. & Ashman, T. (2011). Evidence-based cognitive rehabilitation: Updated review of the literature from 2003 through 2008. *Archives of Physical and Medical Rehabilitation*, 92, 519–530.

Cooper, J. & Malley, D. (2008). *Managing fatigue after brain injury*. Nottingham: Headway.

Cope, N. (1994). Traumatic brain injury rehabilitation outcomes studies in the United States. In A.L. Christensen and B.P. Uzell (eds), *Brain injury and neuropsychological rehabilitation: International perspectives*. Hillsdale, NJ: Lawrence Erlbaum Associates.

Cope, D.N., Cole, J.R., Hall, K.M. & Barkan, H. (1991). Brain injury: Analysis of outcome in a post-acute rehabilitation system. *Brain Injury*, 5, 111–139.

Crosson, B., Barco, P.P., Vallejo, C.A., Bolesta, M.M., Cooper, P.V., Werts, D. & Brobeck, T.C. (1989). Awareness of compensation in post acute head injury rehabilitation. *Journal of Head Trauma Rehabilitation, 4*, 46–54.

Darolles, M. (1875). Ramollissement des protubérances: thrombose du tronc basilaire. *Progress in Medicine, 3*(629).

DiClemente, C.C. & Prochaska, J.O. (1982). Self change and therapy change of smoking behavior: A comparison of processes of change in cessation and maintenance. *Addictive Behavior, 7*, 133–142.

Diller, L.L. (1976). A model for cognitive retraining in rehabilitation. *The Clinical Psychologist, 29*, 13–15.

Doble, J.E., Haig, A.J., Anderson, C. & Katz, R. (2003). Impairment, activity, participation, life satisfaction, and survival in persons with locked-in syndrome for over a decade: Follow-up on a previously reported cohort. *The Journal of Head Trauma Rehabilitation, 18*, 435–444.

Dumas, A. (1844[1846]). *The Count of Monte Cristo.* [Le Comte de Monte Cristo] *Journal des Débats*, France [English trans. (1846). Chapman and Hall].

Duncan J. (1986). Disorganisation of behaviour after frontal lobe damage. *Cognitive Neuropsychology, 3*, 271–290.

Ehlers, A. & Clark, D.M. (2000). A cognitive model of posttraumatic stress disorder. *Journal of Behaviour Research and Therapy, 38*, 319–345.

Enteria, R. & Florschutz, G. (2012). Integrated interdisciplinary team approaches between anthroposophic and conventional medicine: An effective rehabilitation treatment programme in the recovery of a minimally conscious patient following TB meningitis. Poster presented at the 9th international meeting of the WFNR Special Interest Group in Neuropsychological Rehabilitation, Bergen, Norway.

Evans, J.J., Greenfield, E., Wilson, B.A. & Bateman, A. (2009). Walking and talking therapy: Improving cognitive-motor dual tasking in neurological illness. *Journal of International Neuropsychological Society, 15*(1), 112–120.

Fleming, J.M. & Ownsworth, T. (2006). A review of awareness interventions in brain injury rehabilitation. *Neuropsychological Rehabilitation, 16*(4), 474–500.

Fleminger, S., Oliver, D.L., Williams, W.H. & Evans, J.J. (2003). The neuropsychiatry of depression after brain injury. *Neuropsychological Rehabilitation, 13*, 65–87.

Garg, R.K. (2010). Tuberculous meningitis. *Acta Neurologica Scandinavica, 122*, 75–90.

Garrard, P., Bradshaw, D., Jäger, H.R., Thompson, A.J., Losseff, N. & Playford, D. (2002). Cognitive dysfunction after isolated brain stem insult: An underdiagnosed cause of long term morbidity. *Journal of Neurology, Neurosurgery, & Psychiatry.* August, *73*(2), 191–194.

Gilbert, P. (2000). Social mentalities: Internal 'social' conflicts and the role of inner warmth and compassion in cognitive therapy. In P. Gilbert and K.G. Bailey (eds), *Genes on the couch: Explorations in evolutionary psychotherapy* (pp. 118–150). Hove, UK: Brunner-Routledge.

Gilbert, P. (2005). *Compassion: Conceptualisations, research and use in psychotherapy*. Hove, UK: Routledge.

Gilbert, P. (2009). *The compassionate mind*. London: Constable & Robinson.

Gilbert, P. (2010a). *Compassion focused therapy: Distinctive features*. London: Routledge.

Gilbert P. (ed.). (2010b). Compassion focused therapy [Special issue]. *International Journal of Cognitive Therapy*, *3*(2), 95–210.

Gilbert, P. & Irons, C. (2005). Focused therapies and compassionate mind training for shame and self-attacking. In P. Gilbert (ed.), *Compassion: Conceptualisations, research and use in psychotherapy* (pp. 263–325). Hove, UK: Routledge.

Golding E. (1989). MEAMS: The Middlesex elderly assessment of mental state. Titchfield: Thames Valley Test Co.

Gracey, F. & Ownsworth, T. (2008). The self and identity in rehabilitation – editorial *Neuropsychological Rehabilitation*, *18*, 522–526.

Gracey, F., Palmer, S., Rous, B., Psaila, K., Shaw, K., O'Dell, J., Cope, J. & Mohamed, S. (2008). 'Feeling part of things': Personal construction of self after brain injury. *Neuropsychological Rehabilitation*, *18*, 5–6.

Greenwood, R.J. & McMillan, T.M. (1993). Models of rehabilitation programmes for the brain-injured adult – II: Model services and suggestions for change in the UK. *Clinical Rehabilitation*, *7*, 346–355.

Hammond, C. (2010, September 10). Health Check: Art Therapy for Brain Injury Patients [video format]. Retrieved from http://bbc.co.uk/news/health-11265289.

Hart, T., Fann, J.R. & Novack, T.A. (2008). The dilemma of the control condition in experience-based cognitive and behavioural treatment research *Neuropsychological Rehabilitation*, *18*, 1–21.

Henderson, L. (2011). *The compassionate-mind guide to building social confidence: Using Compassion-Focused Therapy to overcome shyness and social anxiety*. Oakland, CA: New Harbinger Publications.

Kabat-Zinn, J. (2005). *Coming to our senses: Healing ourselves and the world through mindfulness* (p. 606). New York: Hyperion.

Kielhofner, G., Braveman, B., Baron, K., Fisher, G., Hammel, J. & Littleton, M. (1999). The model of human occupation: Understanding the worker who is injured or disabled. *Work*, *12*(1), 37–45.

Kolb, D. A., Boyatzis, R. E. & Mainemelis, C. (2001). Experiential learning theory: Previous research and new directions. *Perspectives on thinking, learning, and cognitive styles*, *1*, 227–247.

Kumar, R., Prakash, M., Jha, S. (2006). Paradoxical response to chemotherapy in neurotuberculosis. *Pediatric Neurosurgery*, *42*, 214–222.

Lambert, M. J. & Barley, D. E. (2001). Research summary on the therapeutic relationship and psychotherapy outcome. *Psychotherapy: Theory, Research, Practice, Training*, *38*(4), 357–361.

Laureys, S., Pellas, F., Van Eeckhout, P., Ghorbel, S., Schnakers, C., Perrin, F., Berré, J., Faymonville, M., Pantke, K., Damas, F., *et al.* (2005). The locked-in syndrome: What is it like to be conscious but paralyzed and voiceless? *Progress in Brain Research*, 150, 495–511.

Law, M., Baptiste, S., McColl, M., Opzoomer, A., Polatajko, H. & Pollock, H. (1990). The Canadian occupational performance measure: An outcome measure for occupational therapy. *Canadian Journal of Occupational Therapy*, *57*(2), 82–87.

Lee, D. (2005). The perfect nurturer. A model to develop a compassionate mind within the context of cognitive therapy. In P. Gilbert (ed.), *Compassion: Conceptualisations, research and use in psychotherapy* (pp. 326–351). Hove, UK: Routledge.

Levine, B., Robertson, I.H., Clare, L., Carter, G., Hong, J., Wilson, B.A., Duncan, J. & Stuss, D.T. (2000). Rehabilitation of executive functioning: An experimental-clinical validation of Goal Management Training. *Journal of the International Neuropsychological Society*, *6*, 299–312.

Lima, M.A., Maranhao-Filho, P., Dobbin, J., Apa, A.G., Lima, G.A., Velasco, E. & Sant'anna, C.C. (2012). Paradoxical worsening of brain tuberculomas during treatment. *Archives of Neurology*, *69*(1), 138–139.

MacNiven, J.A., Poz, R., Bainbridge, K., Gracey, F. & Wilson, B.A. (2003). Case study: Emotional adjustment following cognitive recovery from 'persistent vegetative state': Psychological and personal perspectives. *Brain Injury*, *17*(6), 525–533.

Malley, D. & Cooper, J. (2006). *Formulating fatigue in a cognitive-behavioural framework*. Unpublished.

Mehlbye, J. & Larsen, A. (1994). Social and economic consequences of brain damage in Denmark. In A.L. Christensen and B.P. Uzell (eds), *Brain injury and neuropsychological rehabilitation: International perspectives* (pp. 257–267). Hillsdale, NJ: Lawrence Erlbaum Associates.

Miller, W. & Rollnick, S. (2012). *Motivational interviewing: Helping people change (applications of motivational interviewing)* (3rd edn). New York: Guilford Press.

Miotto, E., Evans, J.J., Souza de Lucia, M.C. & Scaff, M. (2009). Rehabilitation of executive dysfunction: A controlled trial of an attention and problem solving treatment group. *Neuropsychological Rehabilitation*, *19*, 517–540.

Misra, U.K., Kalita, J. & Maurya, P.K. (2011). Stroke in tuberculous meningitis. *Journal of Neurological Sciences*, *15*, 22–30.

New, P.W. & Thomas, S.J. (2005). Cognitive impairments in the locked-in syndrome: A case report. *Archives of Physical Medicine and Rehabilitation*, February, *86*(2), 338–343.

Oddy, M. & Herbert, C. (2003). Intervention with families following brain injury: Evidence-based practice. *Neuropsychological Rehabilitation*, *13*, 1–2, 259–273.

Pauk, W. & Owens, R. (2007). *How to study in college*. Boston, MA: Houghton Mifflin.

Posner, M.I. & Peterson, S.E. (1990). The attention system of the human brain. *Annual Review of Neuroscience*, *13*, 25–42.

Post-traumatic stress disorder (PTSD): the treatment of PTSD in adults and children (2005). The National Institute for Clinical Excellence, the Department of Health. Retrieved from http://nice.org.uk/nicemedia/pdf/CG026publicinfo. pdf on 12 September 2012.

Prigatano, G.P. (1986). Personality and psychosocial consequences of brain injury. In G.P. Prigatano, D.J. Fordyce, H.K. Zeiner, J.R. Roueche, M. Pepping and B.C. Wood (eds), *Neuropsychological rehabilitation after brain injury*. Baltimore; London: The Johns Hopkins University Press.

Prigatano, G.P. (1999). *Principles of neuropsychological rehabilitation*. New York: Oxford University Press.

Prigatano, G. (2005). Disturbances of self-awareness and rehabilitation of patients with traumatic brain injury: A 20-year perspective. *Journal of Head Trauma Rehabilitation*, *20*, 1, 19–29.

Prigatano, G. & Pliskin, N.H. (eds). (2002). *Clinical neuropsychology and cost-outcome research: An introduction* (pp. 329–349). Hove, UK: Psychology Press.

Prince, L. & Ford, C. (2012). Can alexithymia be improved? Poster presentation, Symposium at 9th World Congress Satellite Symposium for NeuroRehabilitation. Bergen: Norway.

Robertson, I.H. (1996). *Goal management training: A clinical manual*. Cambridge: PsyConsult.

Robertson, I.H, Ward, T., Ridgeway, V. & Nimmo-Smith, I. (1994). *The Test of Everyday Attention (TEA)*. Bury St Edmunds: Thames Valley Test Company.

Sancisi, E., Battistini, A., Di Stefano, C., Simoncini, L., Montagna, P. & Piperno, R. (2009). Late recovery from post-traumatic vegetative state. *Brain Injury*, *23*, 163–166.

Sarà, M., Sacco, S., Cipolla, F., Onorati, P., Scoppetta, C., Albertini, G. & Carolei, A. (2007). An unexpected recovery from permanent vegetative state. *Brain Injury*, *21*(1),101–103.

Schnakers, C., Majerus, S., Goldman, S., Boly, M., Van Eeckhout, P., Gay, S., Pellas, F., Bartsch, V., Peigneux, P., Moonen, G. *et al.* (2008). Cognitive function in the locked-in syndrome. *Journal of Neurology*, March, *255*(3), 323–330.

Shiel, A., Wilson, B.A., McLellan, L., Horn, S. & Watson, M. (2000). *The Wessex Head Injury Matrix (WHIM)*. Bury St Edmunds: Thames Valley Test Company.

Smith, E. & Delargy, M. (2005). Clinical review: Locked-in syndrome. *British Medical Journal*, *330*, 406–409.

Sopena, S., Dewar, B.K., Nannery, R., Teasdale, T.W. & Wilson, B.A. (2007). The European Brain Injury Questionnaire (EBIQ) as a reliable outcome measure for use with people with brain injury. *Brain Injury*, *21*(10), 1063–1068.

Stern, Y. (2007). *Cognitive reserve: Theory and applications*. New York: Taylor & Francis.

Sterr, A., Herron, K.A., Hayward, C. & Montaldi, D. (2006). Are mild head injuries as mild as we think? Neurobehavioral concomitants of chronic post-concussion syndrome. *BMC Neurology*, *6*(1), 7.

Swihart, A.A., Boller, F., Saxton, J. & McGonigle, K.L. (1993). *The Severe Impairment Battery*. London: Pearson Assessment UK.

Tavalaro, J. & Tayson, R. (1997). *Look up for yes*. New York: Ko-dansha America Inc.

Teasdale, T.W., Emslie, H., Quirk, K., Evans, J.J., Fish, J. & Wilson, B.A. (2009). Alleviation of carer strain during the use of the NeuroPage device by people with acquired brain injury. *Journal of Neurology, Neurosurgery & Psychiatry*, *80*, 781–783.

Teasdale, T.W. & Engberg, A.W. (2001). Suicide after traumatic brain injury: A population study. *Journal of Neurology, Neurosurgery & Psychiatry*, *71*, 436–440.

Tyerman, A. & Booth, J. (2001). Family interventions after traumatic brain injury: A service example. *Neuropsychological Rehabilitation*, *16*, 59–66.

Van Heugten, C., Gregório, G.W. & Wade, D. (2012). Evidence-based cognitive rehabilitation after acquired brain injury: A systematic review of content of treatment. *Neuropsychological Rehabilitation*, *22*, 653–673.

Victor, M., Adams, R.D. & Collins, G.H. (1989). *The Wernicke-Korsakoff Syndrome* (2nd edn). Philadelphia, PA: FA Davis Co.

Vigand, P. & Vigand, S. (2000). *Only the eyes say yes* (original title: *Putain de silence*). New York: Arcade Publishing.

Von Cramon, D.M., Matthes-von Cramon, G. & Mai, N. (1991). Problem-solving deficits in brain-injured patients: A therapeutic approach. *Neuropsychological Rehabilitation*, *1*, 45–64.

Waters, F. & Bucks, R.S. (2011). Neuropsychological effects of sleep loss: Implication for neuropsychologists. *Journal of the International Neuropsychological Society*, *17*, 571–586.

Wells, A. (2008). *Metacognitive therapy for anxiety and depression*. New York: Guilford Press. (Contains the ATT treatment manual for therapists.)

Wells, A. & Matthews, G. (1994). *Attention and emotion: A clinical perspective*. Hove, UK: Psychology Press.

West, M., Wehman, P., Kregel, J., Kreutzer, J., Sherron, P. & Zasler, N. (1991). Costs of operating a supported work program for traumatically brain-injured individuals. *Archives of Physical Medicine and Rehabilitation*, *72*, 127–131.

White, M. & Epston, D. (1990). *Narrative means to therapeutic ends*. New York: W.W. Norton.

Whyte, J. (1997). Assessing medical rehabilitation practices: Distinctive methodologic challenges. In M.J. Fuhrer (ed.), *The promises of outcomes research* (pp. 43–59). Baltimore, MD: Paul Brookes Publishing Company.

Williams, M. & Smith, H.V. (1954). Mental disturbances in tuberculous meningitis. *Journal of Neurology, Neurosurgery & Psychiatry, 17*, 173–182.

Wilson, B.A. (2002). Towards a comprehensive model of cognitive rehabilitation. *Neuropsychological Rehabilitation, 12*, 97–110.

Wilson, B.A. (2009). Kate: cognitive recovery and emotional adjustment in a young woman who was unresponsive for several months. In B.A. Wilson, F. Gracey, J.J. Evans & A. Bateman, *Neuropsychological rehabilitation: Theory, models, therapy and outcomes*. Cambridge: Cambridge University Press.

Wilson, B.A., Baddeley, A., Evans, J. & Shiel, A. (1994). Errorless learning in the rehabilitation of memory impaired people. *Neuropsychological Rehabilitation, 3*(4), 307–326

Wilson, B.A., Emslie, H.C., Quirk, K. & Evans, J.J. (2001). Reducing everyday memory and planning problems by means of a paging system: A randomised control crossover study. *Journal of Neurology, Neurosurgery & Psychiatry, 70*(4), 477–482.

Wilson, B.A. & Evans, J.J. (2002). Does cognitive rehabilitation work? Clinical and economic considerations and outcomes. In G. Prigatano and N.H. Pliskin (Eds), *Clinical neuropsychology and cost-outcome research: An introduction* (pp. 329–349). Hove, UK: Psychology Press.

Wilson, B.A., Gracey, F. & Bainbridge, K. (2001). Cognitive recovery from 'persistent vegetative state': Psychological and personal perspectives. *Brain Injury, 15*, 1083–1092.

Wilson, B.A., Gracey, F., Evans, J.J. & Bateman, A. (2009). *Neuropsychological rehabilitation: Theory, models, therapy and outcomes*. Cambridge: Cambridge University Press.

Wilson, B.A., Hinchcliffe, A., Kapur, N., Tunnard, C. & Florschutz, G. (in press). Paradoxical recovery more than two years after onset of tuberculous meningitis: A case study. *Brain Injury*.

Wilson, B.A., Hinchcliffe, A., Okines, T., Florschutz, G. & Fish, J. (2011). A case study of locked-in syndrome: Psychological and personal perspectives. *Brain Injury, 25*, 526–538.

Winegardner, J. & Ashworth, F. (2012). The health economy of holistic rehabilitation: Four case studies. Paper presented at the 9th Conference of the Neuropsychological Rehabilitation Special Interest Group of the World Federation of Neurological Rehabilitation, Bergen, Norway.

Winkens, I., Van Heugten, C.M., Wade, D.T., Habets, E.J. & Fasotti, L. (2009). Efficacy of time pressure management in stroke patients with slowed information processing: A randomized controlled trial. *Archives of Physical Medicine and Rehabilitation, 90*(10), 1672–1679.

Winson, R., Saez-Martin, M., Brentnall, S. & Malley, D. (2012). Feeling Understood: Application of The Model Of Human Occupation (MOHO) to Vocational Rehabilitation. Poster presented at the international conference of the International Brain Injury Association in Edinburgh, Scotland.

Wood, R.L., McCrea, J.D., Wood, L.M. & Merriman, R.N. (1999). Clinical and cost effectiveness of post-acute neurobehavioural rehabilitation. *Brain Injury*, *13*, 69–88.

Zigmond, A.S. & Snaith, R.P. (1983). The hospital anxiety and depression scale. *Acta Psychiatrica Scandinavica*, *67*(6), 361–370.

Index

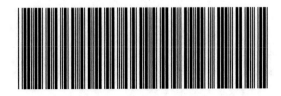